# KALORIK MA
# Air Fryer Oven
# COOKBOOK

## Delicious, Fast and Easy to
## Make Healthy Recipes
## in Your Air Fryer Oven for Beginners

## Includes 50 Super Fast "5 Minutes" Ideas

# TABLE OF CONTENTS

# POULTRY RECIPES

# VEGGIE RECIPES

SEASONED VEGGIES
POTATO GRATIN
BUTTERED BROCCOLI
GARLIC EDAMAME
PESTO GNOCCHI
SPICY CHICKPEAS
CRISP & SPICY CABBAGE
EGG ROLL PIZZA STICKS
CAULIFLOWER RICE
BALSAMIC KALE
CAJUN ZUCCHINI CHIPS
CREAMY CABBAGE
CINNAMON AND SUGAR PEACHES
SPICY CABBAGE
SPICY BROCCOLI WITH HOT SAUCE
CHEESY BROCCOLI GRATIN
COCONUT OIL ARTICHOKES
ROSTI (SWISS POTATOES)
ZUCCHINI CURRY
VEGGIES ON TOAST
JUMBO STUFFED MUSHROOMS
HEALTHY CARROT FRIES
SIMPLE ROASTED CARROTS
BROCCOLI & CHEESE
PARMESAN ASPARAGUS FRIES
CAULIFLOWER HASH
SWEET POTATO & ONION MIX
AIR FRIED ROASTED CORN ON THE COB
CHILI BROCCOLI
AIR FRIED HONEY ROASTED CARROTS
AIR FRIED ROASTED CABBAGE
CARAMELIZED BROCCOLI
BRUSSELS SPROUTS WITH BALSAMIC OIL
SHREDDED CABBAGE
CHARRED GREEN BEANS WITH SEEDS

# FISH & SEAFOOD

CHEESY LEMON HALIBUT
SHRIMP CROQUETTES
SPICY MACKEREL
THYME SCALLOPS
BUTTERY SHRIMP SKEWERS

Mustard Salmon
Chinese Style Cod
Salmon and Orange Marmalade
Tilapia & Chives Sauce
Marinated Salmon Recipe
Tasty Grilled Red Mullet
Cajun Salmon
Garlicky-Grilled Turbot
Char-Grilled Spicy Halibut
Swordfish with Charred Leeks
Breaded Coconut Shrimp
Cod Fish Nuggets
Grilled Sardines
Fried Catfish
Creamy Salmon
Crumbled Fish
Easy Crab Sticks
Deep Fried Prawns
Zucchini with Tuna
Caramelized Salmon Fillet
Mussels with Pepper
Monkfish with Olives and Capers
Shrimp, Zucchini and Cherry Tomato
Salted Marinated Salmon
Salmon with Pistachio Bark
Sautéed Trout with Almonds
Air Fryer Shrimp a La Bang
Breaded Cod Sticks
Air Fried Crumbed Fish
Rabas
Honey Glazed Salmon
Sweet & Sour Glazed Salmon

# DESSERT
Coconut Donuts
Apple Chips
Blueberry Cream
Blackberry Chia Jam
Mixed Berries Cream
Cinnamon-Spiced Acorn Squash
Sweetened Plantains
Pear Crisp

## SUPER FAST 5-MINUTES RECIPES

## CONCLUSION

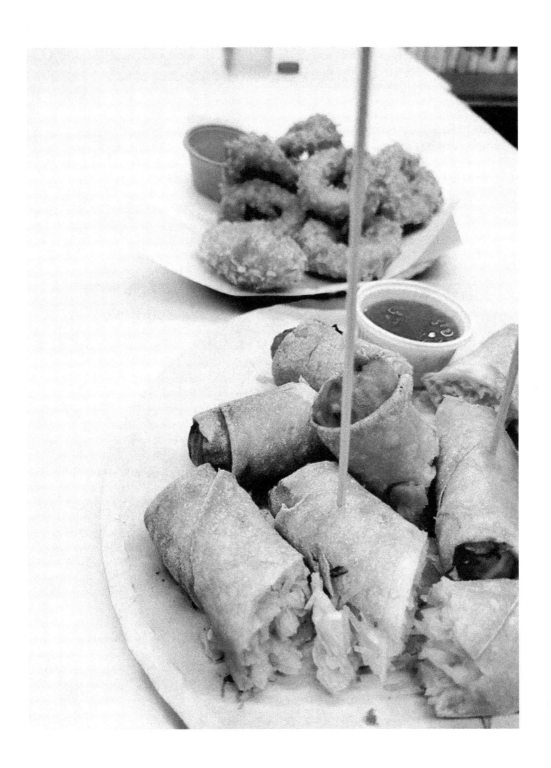

# Introduction

The Kalorik Maxx Air Fryer Oven is an "all-in-one" kitchen appliance that promises **to replace a deep fryer, convection oven and microwave**; it also lets you sauté your foods. The Kalorik Maxx Air Fryer Oven is a unique kitchen gadget designed to fry food in a special chamber using super-heated air. In fact, the hot air circulates inside the cooking chamber using the convection mechanism, cooking your food evenly from all sides. It uses the so-called Maillard effect – a chemical reaction that gives fried food that distinctive flavor. Simply put, thanks to the hot air, your foods get that crispy exterior and a moist interior and does not taste like the fat.

Why use an Air Fryer? I'm asked this question time and time again, so my answer is always the same: it all boils down to **versatility**, **health**, and **speed**. It means that you can "set it and forget it" until it is done. Unlike most cooking methods, there's no need to keep an eye on it. **You can pick the ingredients, turn the machine on and walk away** – no worries about overcooked or burned food. Another great benefit of using an Air Fryer is that unlike the heat in your oven or on a stovetop, the heat in the cooking chamber is constant and it allows your food to cook evenly. Plus, it is an energy-efficient and space-saving solution.

Air fryers operate by cooking food with the flow of hot air. This is what makes the foods you put into it so crunchy when they come out! This is what makes the foods you put into it so crunchy when they come out! There is this thing called the "Maillard Effect" that happens, which is a chemically prompted reaction that happens to the high temperature that makes it proficient for this fryer to cook foods in such little time while the nutrients and flavor are intact.

# Benefits of the Air Fryer

There are numerous benefits you'll get from using an Air Fryer. Here are the top three benefits of using an Air Fryer.

### Fast cooking and convenience

The Kalorik Maxx Air Fryer Oven is an electric device, so you just need to press the right buttons and go about your business. It heats up in a few minutes so it can cut down cooking time; further, hot air circulates around your food, cooking it quickly and evenly. **Roast chicken is perfectly cooked in 30 minutes, baby back ribs in less than 25 minutes and beef chuck or steak in about 15 minutes**. You can use dividers and cook different foods at the same time. The Air Fryer is a real game-changer, it is a cost-saving solution in many ways. I also use my Air Fryer to keep my food warm. Air Fryer features include automatic temperature control, eliminating the need to slave over a hot stove.

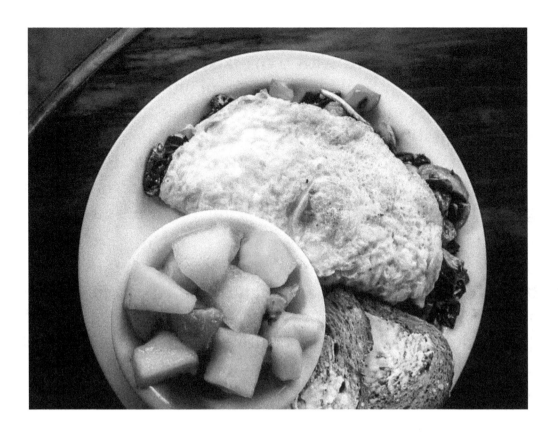

**Healthy eating**. Yes, there is such a thing as healthy fried food and the Air Fryer proves that! The Air Fryer inspires me every day so that I enjoy cooking healthy and well-balanced meals for my family. Recent studies have shown that **air-fried foods contain up to 80% less fat in comparison to foods that are deep-fried**. Deep-fried food contributes to obesity, type 2 diabetes, high cholesterol, increased risk of heart disease, and so on. Plus, fats and oils become harmful under the high heat, which leads to increased inflammation in your body and speeds up aging. Further, these oils release cancer-causing toxic chemicals. Moreover, the spills of fats and oils injure wildlife and produce other undesirable effects on the planet Earth.

According to the leading experts, **you should not be afraid of healthy fats and oils, especially if you follow the ketogenic diet.** Avoid partially hydrogenated and genetically modified oils such as cottonseed oil, soybean oil, corn oil, and rice bran oil. You should also avoid margarine since it is loaded with trans-fats. Good fats and oils include olive oil, coconut oil, avocado oil, sesame oil, nuts and seeds. **Air-fried foods are delicious and have the texture of regular fried food, but they do not taste like fat**. French fries are only the beginning. Perfect ribs, hearty casseroles, fast snacks, and delectable desserts turn out great in this revolutionary kitchen gadget. When it comes to healthy dieting that does not compromise flavor, the Air Fryer is a real winner.

**The ultimate solution to losing pounds and maintain a healthy weight.** One of the greatest benefits of owning an Air Fryer is **the possibility to maintain an ideal weight in an easy and healthy way**. It doesn't mean that you must give up fried fish fillets, saucy steaks, and scrumptious desserts. Choosing a healthy-cooking technique is the key to success. Air frying requires less fat compared to many other cooking methods, making your weight loss diet more achievable.

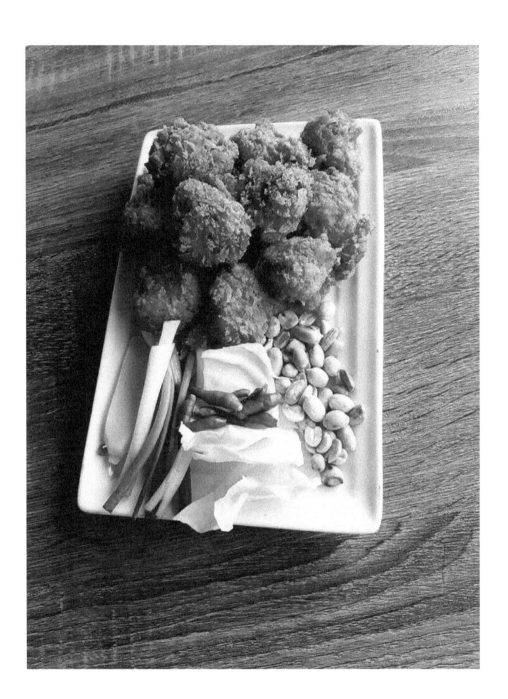

# Breakfast

## Simple Egg Soufflé

**Preparation Time:** 5 minutes | **Cooking Time:** 8 minutes | **Serves:** 2

**Ingredients:**

- 2 eggs
- 1/4 tsp chili pepper
- 2 tbsp heavy cream
- 1/4 tsp pepper
- 1 tbsp parsley, chopped
- Salt

**Directions:**

1. In a bowl, whisk eggs with remaining ingredients.
2. Spray two ramekins with cooking spray.
3. Pour egg mixture into the prepared ramekins and place into your Kalorik Maxx Air Fryer.
4. Cook soufflé at 390°F for 8 minutes
5. Serve and enjoy.

Cal 116 | Fat 10g | Carb 1.1g | Protein 6 g

## Air-Fried English Breakfast

**Preparation Time:** 5 minutes | **Cooking Time:** 20 minutes | **Serves:** 4

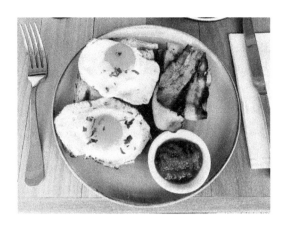

**Ingredients:**

- 8 sausages
- 8 bacon slices
- 4 eggs
- 1 (16-ounce) can of baked beans
- 8 slices of toast

**Directions:**

1. Add the sausages and bacon slices to your air fryer and cook them for 10 minutes at a 320°F.
2. Using a ramekin or heat-safe bowl, add the baked beans, then place another ramekin and add the eggs and whisk.
3. Change the temperature to 290°F.
4. Place it inside your air fryer and cook it for an additional 10 minutes or until everything is done.
5. Serve and enjoy!

Cal 850 | Fat 40g | Carb 20g | Protein 48g

# Sausage and Egg Breakfast Burrito

**Preparation Time:** 5 minutes | **Cooking Time:** 30 minutes | **Serves:** 6

**Ingredients:**

- 6 eggs
- Salt
- Pepper
- Cooking oil

- ½ cup chopped red bell pepper
- ½ cup chopped green bell pepper
- 8 ounces ground chicken sausage
- ½ cup salsa
- 6 medium (8-inch) flour tortillas
- ½ cup shredded Cheddar cheese

**Directions:**

1. In a medium bowl, whisk the eggs. Add salt and pepper to taste.
2. Place a skillet on medium-high heat. Spray with cooking oil. Add the eggs. Scramble for 2 to 3 minutes, until the eggs are fluffy. Remove the eggs from the skillet and set aside.
3. If needed, spray the skillet with more oil. Add the chopped red and green bell peppers. Cook for 2 to 3 minutes, once the peppers are soft.
4. Add the ground sausage to the skillet. Break the sausage into smaller pieces using a spatula or spoon. Cook for 3 to 4 minutes, until the sausage is brown.
5. Add the salsa and scrambled eggs. Stir to combine. Remove the skillet from heat.
6. Spoon the mixture evenly onto the tortillas.
7. To form the burritos, fold the sides of each tortilla in toward the middle and then roll up from the bottom. You can secure each burrito with a toothpick. Or you can moisten the outside edge of the tortilla with a small amount of water. I prefer to use a cooking brush, but you can also dab with your fingers.
8. Spray the burritos with cooking oil and place them in the air fryer. Do not stack. Cook the burritos in batches if they do not all fit in the basket. Cook for 8 minutes
9. Open the air fryer and flip the burritos. Heat it for an additional 2 minutes or until crisp.
10. If necessary, repeat steps 8 and 9 for the remaining burritos.
11. Sprinkle the Cheddar cheese over the burritos. Cool before serving.

Cal 236 | Fat 13g | Carb 16g | Protein 15g

# French Toast Sticks

**Preparation Time:** 5 minutes | **Cooking Time:** 15 minutes | **Serves:** 12

**Ingredients:**

- 4 slices Texas toast (or any thick bread, such as challah)
- 1 tablespoon butter
- 1 egg
- 1 teaspoon stevia
- 1 teaspoon ground cinnamon
- ¼ cup milk
- 1 teaspoon vanilla extract

- Cooking oil

**Directions:**

1. Cut each slice of bread into 3 pieces (for 12 sticks total).
2. Place the butter in a small, microwave-safe bowl. Heat for 15 seconds, or until the butter has melted.
3. Remove the bowl from the microwave. Add the egg, stevia, cinnamon, milk, and vanilla extract. Whisk until fully combined.
4. Sprinkle the air fryer with cooking oil.
5. Dredge each of the bread sticks in the egg mixture.
6. Place the French toast sticks in the air fryer. It is okay to stack them. Spray the French toast sticks with cooking oil. Cook for 8 minutes
7. Open the air fryer and flip each of the French toast sticks. Cook for an additional 4 minutes, or until the French toast sticks are crisp.
8. Cool before serving.

Cal 52 | Fat 2g | Carb 7g | Protein 2g

---

# Home-Fried Potatoes

**Preparation Time:** 5 minutes | **Cooking Time:** 25 minutes | **Serves:** 4

**Ingredients:**

- 3 large russet potatoes
- 1 tablespoon canola oil
- 1 tablespoon extra-virgin olive oil
- 1 teaspoon paprika
- Salt
- Pepper
- 1 cup chopped onion
- 1 cup chopped red bell pepper
- 1 cup chopped green bell pepper

**Directions:**

1. Cut the potatoes into ½-inch cubes. Place the potatoes in a large bowl of cold water and allow them to soak for at least 30 minutes, preferably an hour.
2. Dry out the potatoes and wipe thoroughly with paper towels. Return them to the empty bowl.
3. Add the canola and olive oils, paprika, and salt and pepper to flavor. Toss to fully coat the potatoes.
4. Transfer the potatoes to your Kalorik Maxx Air Fryer. Cook for 20 minutes, shaking the air fryer basket every 5 minutes (a total of 4 times).

5. Put the onion and red and green bell peppers to the Air Fryer basket. Fry for an additional 3 to 4 minutes, or until the potatoes are cooked through and the peppers are soft.
6. Cool before serving.

Cal 279 | Fat 8g | Carb 50g | Protein 6g

# Homemade Cherry Breakfast Tarts

**Preparation Time:** 15 minutes | **Cooking Time:** 20 minutes | **Serves:** 6

**Ingredients:**

For the tarts:
- 2 refrigerated piecrusts
- ⅓ Cup cherry preserves
- 1 teaspoon cornstarch
- Cooking oil

For the frosting:
- ½ cup vanilla yogurt
- 1-ounce cream cheese
- 1 teaspoon stevia
- Rainbow sprinkles

**Directions:**

1. To make the tarts:
2. Place the piecrusts on a flat surface. Make use of a knife or pizza cutter, cut each piecrust into 3 rectangles, for 6 in total. (I discard the unused dough left from slicing the edges.)
3. In a small bowl, combine the preserves and cornstarch. Mix well.
4. Scoop 1 tablespoon of the preserve mixture onto the top half of each piece of piecrust.
5. Fold the bottom of each piece up to close the tart. Press along the edges of each tart to seal using the back of a fork.
6. Sprinkle the breakfast tarts with cooking oil and place them in the air fryer. I do not recommend piling the breakfast tarts. They will stick together if piled. You may need to prepare them in two batches. Cook for 10 minutes
7. Allow the breakfast tarts to cool fully before removing from the air fryer.

8. If needed, repeat steps 5 and 6 for the remaining breakfast tarts.
9. To make the frosting:
10. In a small bowl, mix the yogurt, cream cheese, and stevia. Mix well.
11. Spread the breakfast tarts with frosting and top with sprinkles, and serve.

Cal 119 | Fat 4g | Carb 19g | Protein 2g

# Jalapeno Breakfast Muffins

**Preparation Time:** 10 minutes | **Cooking Time:** 15 minutes | **Serves:** 8

**Ingredients:**

- 5 eggs
- 1/3 cup coconut oil, melted
- 2 tsp baking powder
- 3 tbsp erythritol
- 3 tbsp jalapenos, sliced
- 1/4 cup unsweetened coconut milk
- 2/3 cup coconut flour
- 3/4 tsp sea salt

**Directions:**

1. Preheat the air fryer to 325°F.
2. In a large bowl, mix together coconut flour, baking powder, erythritol, and sea salt.
3. Stir in eggs, jalapenos, coconut milk, and coconut oil until well combined.
4. Pour batter into the silicone muffin molds and place into your Kalorik Maxx Air Fryer.
5. Cook muffins for 15 minutes
6. Serve and enjoy.

Cal 125 | Fat 12g | Carb 7g | Protein 3 g

# Asparagus Frittata

**Preparation Time:** 10 minutes | **Cooking Time:** 10 minutes | **Serves:** 4

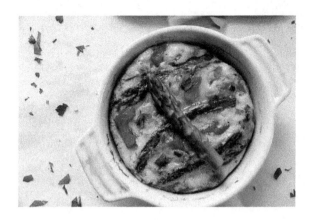

**Ingredients:**
- 6 eggs
- 3 mushrooms, sliced
- 10 asparagus, chopped
- 1/4 cup half and half
- 2 tsp butter, melted
- 1 cup mozzarella cheese, shredded
- 1 tsp pepper
- 1 tsp salt

**Directions:**
1. Toss mushrooms and asparagus with melted butter and add into your Kalorik Maxx Air Fryer. Cook mushrooms and asparagus at 350°F for 5 minutes.
2. Meanwhile, in a bowl, whisk together eggs, half and half, pepper, and salt. Transfer cook mushrooms and asparagus into a proper dish. Pour egg mixture over mushrooms and asparagus.
3. Place dish in the air fryer and cook at 350°F for 5 minutes or until eggs are set. Slice and serve.

Cal 211 | Fat 13g | Carb 4g | Protein 16 g

## Vegetable Egg Soufflé

**Preparation Time:** 10 minutes | **Cooking Time:** 20 minutes | **Serves:** 4

**Ingredients:**
- 4 large eggs
- 1 tsp onion powder
- 1 tsp garlic powder
- 1 tsp red pepper, crushed
- 1/2 cup broccoli florets, chopped

- 1/2 cup mushrooms, chopped

**Directions:**
1. Sprinkle four ramekins with cooking spray and set aside.
2. In a bowl, whisk eggs with onion powder, garlic powder, and red pepper.
3. Add mushrooms and broccoli and stir well.
4. Pour egg mixture into the prepared ramekins and place ramekins into your Kalorik Maxx Air Fryer.
5. Cook at 350°F for 15 minutes. Make sure soufflé is cooked if soufflé is not cooked then cook for 5 minutes more.
6. Serve and enjoy.

Cal 91 | Fat 5.1g | Carb 4.7g | Protein 7.4g

# Spicy Cauliflower Rice

**Preparation Time:** 10 minutes | **Cooking Time:** 22 minutes | **Serves:** 2

**Ingredients:**
- 1 cauliflower head, cut into florets
- 1/2 tsp cumin
- 1/2 tsp chili powder
- 6 onion spring, chopped
- 2 jalapenos, chopped
- 4 tbsp olive oil
- 1 zucchini, trimmed and cut into cubes
- 1/2 tsp paprika
- 1/2 tsp garlic powder
- 1/2 tsp cayenne pepper
- 1/2 tsp pepper
- 1/2 tsp salt

**Directions:**
1. Preheat the air fryer to 370°F.
2. Add cauliflower florets into the food processor and process until it looks like rice.
3. Transfer cauliflower rice into the baking pan and rizzle with half oil.
4. Place pan in the air fryer and cook for 12 minutes, stir halfway through.
5. Heat the remaining oil in a small pan over medium heat.
6. Add zucchini and cook for 5-8 minutes
7. Add onion and jalapenos and cook for 5 minutes
8. Add spices and stir well. Set aside.
9. Add cauliflower rice in the zucchini mixture and stir well.
10. Serve and enjoy.

Cal 254 | Fat 28g | Carb 12g | Protein 4.3 g

# Mushroom Frittata

**Preparation Time:** 10 minutes | **Cooking Time:** 13 minutes | **Serves:** 1

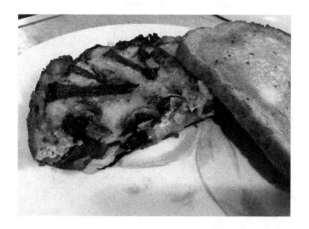

**Ingredients:**
- 1 cup egg whites
- 1 cup spinach, chopped
- 2 mushrooms, sliced
- 2 tbsp parmesan cheese, grated
- Salt

**Directions:**
1. Sprinkle pan with cooking spray and heat over medium heat. Add mushrooms and sauté for 2-3 minutes. Add spinach and cook for 1-2 minutes or until wilted.
2. Transfer mushroom spinach mixture into the baking pan. Beat egg whites in a mixing bowl until frothy. Season it with a pinch of salt.
3. Pour egg white mixture into the spinach and mushroom mixture and sprinkle with parmesan cheese. Place pan in air fryer and cook frittata at 350°F for 8 minutes
4. Slice and serve.

Cal 176 | Fat 3g | Carb 4g | Protein 31 g

# Broccoli Stuffed Peppers

**Preparation Time:** 10 minutes | **Cooking Time:** 40 minutes | **Serves:** 2

**Ingredients:**
- 4 eggs
- 1/2 cup cheddar cheese, grated

- 2 bell peppers cut in half and remove seeds
- 1/2 tsp garlic powder
- 1 tsp dried thyme
- 1/4 cup feta cheese, crumbled
- 1/2 cup broccoli, cooked
- 1/4 tsp pepper
- 1/2 tsp salt

**Directions:**
1. Preheat the air fryer to 325°F.
2. Stuff feta and broccoli into the bell peppers halved.
3. Beat egg in a bowl with seasoning and pour egg mixture into the pepper halved over feta and broccoli.
4. Place bell pepper halved into your Kalorik Maxx Air Fryer and cook for 35-40 minutes
5. Top with grated cheddar cheese and cook until cheese melted.
6. Serve and enjoy.

Cal 340 | Fat 22g | Carb 12g | Protein 22 g

# Zucchini Noodles

**Preparation Time:** 10 minutes | **Cooking Time:** 44 minutes | **Serves:** 3

**Ingredients:**
- 1 egg
- 1/2 cup parmesan cheese, grated
- 1/2 cup feta cheese, crumbled
- 1 tbsp thyme
- 1 garlic clove, chopped
- 1 onion, chopped
- 2 medium zucchinis, trimmed and spiralized
- 2 tbsp olive oil
- 1 cup mozzarella cheese, grated
- 1/2 tsp pepper
- 1/2 tsp salt

**Directions:**
1. Preheat the air fryer to 350°F.
2. Add spiralized zucchini and salt in a colander and set aside for 10 minutes. Wash zucchini noodles and pat dry with a paper towel.
3. Heat the oil in a pan over medium heat. Add garlic and onion and sauté for 3-4 minutes
4. Add zucchini noodles and cook for 4-5 minutes or until softened.

5. Add zucchini mixture into the baking pan. Add egg, thyme, cheeses. Mix well and season.
6. Place pan in the air fryer and cook for 30-35 minutes
7. Serve and enjoy

Cal 435 | Fat 29g | Carb 10g | Protein 25 g

---

## Egg Muffins

**Preparation Time:** 10 minutes | **Cooking Time:** 15 minutes | **Serves:** 12

**Ingredients:**

- 9 eggs
- 1/2 cup onion, sliced
- 1 tbsp olive oil
- 8 oz ground sausage
- 1/4 cup coconut milk
- 1/2 tsp oregano
- 1 1/2 cups spinach
- 3/4 cup bell peppers, chopped
- Pepper
- Salt

**Directions:**

1. Preheat the air fryer to 325°F.
2. Add ground sausage in a pan and sauté over medium heat for 5 minutes
3. Add olive oil, oregano, bell pepper, and onion and sauté until onion is translucent.
4. Put spinach to the pan and cook for 30 seconds.
5. Remove pan from heat and set aside.
6. In a mixing bowl, whisk together eggs, coconut milk, pepper, and salt until well beaten.
7. Add sausage and vegetable mixture into the egg mixture and mix well.
8. Pour egg mixture into the silicone muffin molds and place into your Kalorik Maxx Air Fryer. (Cook in batches)
9. Cook muffins for 15 minutes
10. Serve and enjoy.

Cal 135 | Fat 11g | Carb 1.5g | Protein 8 g

---

## Yummy Breakfast
## Italian Frittata

**Preparation Time:** 5 minutes | **Cooking Time:** 10 minutes | **Serves:** 6

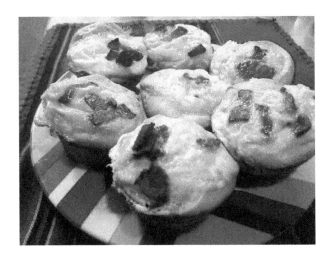

**Ingredients:**

- 6 eggs
- 1/3 cup of milk
- 4-ounces of chopped Italian sausage
- 3 cups of stemmed and roughly chopped kale
- 1 red deseeded and chopped bell pepper
- ½ cup of a grated feta cheese
- 1 chopped zucchini
- 1 tablespoon of freshly chopped basil
- 1 teaspoon of garlic powder
- 1 teaspoon of onion powder
- 1 teaspoon of salt
- 1 teaspoon of black pepper

**Directions:**

1. Turn on your air fryer to 360°F.
2. Grease the air fryer pan with a nonstick cooking spray.
3. Add the Italian sausage to the pan and cook it inside your air fryer for 5 minutes
4. While doing that, add and stir in the remaining ingredients until it mixes properly.
5. Add the egg mixture to the pan and allow it to cook inside your air fryer for 5 minutes
6. Thereafter carefully remove the pan and allow it to cool off until it gets chill enough to serve.
7. Serve and enjoy!

Cal 225 | Fat 14g | Carb 4.5g | Protein 20g

# Seasoned Potatoes

**Preparation Time:** 5 minutes | **Cooking Time:** 40 minutes | **Serves:** 2

**Ingredients:**
- Russet potatoes – 2, scrubbed
- Butter – ½ tbsp. melted
- Garlic & herb blend seasoning – ½ tsp.
- Garlic powder – ½ tsp.
- Salt, as required

**Directions:**
1. In a bowl, mix all of the spices and salt.
2. With a fork, prick the potatoes. Coat the potatoes with butter and sprinkle with spice mixture.
3. Preheat the air fryer to 400°F.
4. Arrange the potatoes onto the cooking rack, insert the cooking rack in the center position and cook for 40 minutes. Serve hot.

Cal 176 | Carb 34g | Fat 2.1g | Protein 3.8g

# Savory Cheese and Bacon Muffins

**Preparation Time:** 5 minutes | **Cooking Time:** 17 minutes | **Serves:** 4

**Ingredients:**
- 1 ½ cup of all-purpose flour
- 2 teaspoons of baking powder
- ½ cup of milk
- 2 eggs
- 1 tablespoon of freshly chopped parsley
- 4 cooked and chopped bacon slices
- 1 thinly chopped onion
- ½ cup of shredded cheddar cheese
- ½ teaspoon of onion powder
- 1 teaspoon of salt
- 1 teaspoon of black pepper

**Directions:**
1. Turn on your air fryer to 360°F.
2. Using a large bowl, add and stir all the ingredients until it mixes properly.
3. Then grease the muffin cups with a nonstick cooking spray or line it with a parchment paper. Pour the batter proportionally into each muffin cup.

4. Place it inside your air fryer and bake it for 15 minutes
5. Thereafter, carefully remove it from your air fryer and allow it to chill.
6. Serve and enjoy!

Cal 180 | Fat 18g | Carb 16g | Protein 15g

---

# Fried Chicken and Waffles

**Preparation Time:** 10 minutes | **Cooking Time:** 30 minutes | **Serves:** 4

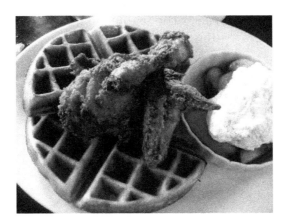

**Ingredients:**

- 8 whole chicken wings
- 1 teaspoon garlic powder
- Chicken seasoning or rub
- Pepper
- ½ cup all-purpose flour
- Cooking oil
- 8 frozen waffles
- Maple syrup (optional)

**Directions:**

1. In a medium bowl, spice the chicken with the garlic powder and chicken seasoning and pepper to flavor.
2. Put the chicken to a sealable plastic bag and add the flour. Shake to thoroughly coat the chicken.
3. Sprinkle the air fryer basket with cooking oil.

4. With the use of tongs, put the chicken from the bag to your Kalorik Maxx Air Fryer. It is okay to pile the chicken wings on top of each other. Sprinkle them with cooking oil. Heat for five minutes
5. Unlock the air fryer and shake the basket. Presume to cook the chicken. Keep shaking every 5 minutes until 20 minutes has passed and the chicken is completely cooked.
6. Take out the cooked chicken from the air fryer and set aside.
7. Wash the basket and base out with warm water. Put them back to the Air Fryer.
8. Ease the temperature of the air fryer to 370ºF.
9. Put the frozen waffles in the air fryer. Do not pile. Depends on how big your air fryer is, you may need to cook the waffles in batches. Sprinkle the waffles with cooking oil. Cook for 6 minutes
10. If necessary, take out the cooked waffles from the air fryer, then repeat step 9 for the leftover waffles.
11. Serve the waffles with the chicken and a bit of maple syrup if desired.

Cal 461 | Fat 22g | Carb 45g | Protein 28g

# Sausage and Cream Cheese Biscuits

**Preparation Time:** 5 minutes | **Cooking Time:** 15 minutes | **Serves:** 5

**Ingredients:**
- 12 ounces chicken breakfast sausage
- 1 (6-ounce) can biscuits
- ⅛ cup cream cheese

**Direction:**
1. Form the sausage into 5 small patties.
2. Place the sausage patties in the air fryer. Cook for 5 minutes
3. Open the air fryer. Flip the patties. Cook for an additional 5 minutes
4. Remove the cooked sausages from the air fryer.
5. Separate the biscuit dough into 5 biscuits.
6. Place the biscuits in the air fryer. Cook for 3 minutes
7. Open the air fryer. Flip the biscuits. Cook for an additional 2 minutes
8. Remove the cooked biscuits from the air fryer.
9. Split each biscuit in half. Spread 1 teaspoon of cream cheese onto the bottom of each biscuit. Top with a sausage patty and the other half of the biscuit, and serve.

Cal 120 | Fat 13g | Carb 7.3g | Protein 9g

# Cheesy Tater Tot Breakfast Bake

**Preparation Time:** 5 minutes | **Cooking Time:** 20 minutes | **Serves:** 4

**Ingredients:**

- 4 eggs
- 1 cup milk
- 1 teaspoon onion powder
- Salt
- Pepper
- Cooking oil
- 12 ounces ground chicken sausage
- 1-pound frozen tater tots
- ¾ cup shredded Cheddar cheese

**Directions:**

1. In a medium bowl, whisk the eggs. Add the milk, onion powder, and salt and pepper to taste. Stir to combine.
2. Spray a skillet with cooking oil and set over medium-high heat. Add the ground sausage. Using a spatula or spoon, break the sausage into smaller pieces. Cook for 3 to 4 minutes, until the sausage is brown. Remove from heat and set aside.
3. Spray a barrel pan with cooking oil. Make sure to cover the bottom and sides of the pan.
4. Place the tater tots in the barrel pan. Cook for 6 minutes
5. Open the air fryer and shake the pan, then add the egg mixture and cooked sausage. Cook for an additional 6 minutes. Open the air fryer and sprinkle the cheese over the tater tot bake. Cook for an additional 2 to 3 minutes.
6. Cool before serving.

Cal 518 | Fat 30g | Carb 31g | Protein 30g

# Breakfast Grilled Ham and Cheese

**Preparation Time:** 5 minutes | **Cooking Time:** 10 minutes | **Serves:** 2

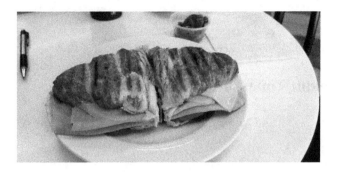

**Ingredients:**

- 1 teaspoon butter
- 4 slices bread
- 4 slices smoked country ham
- 4 slices Cheddar cheese
- 4 thick slices tomato

**Directions:**

1. Spread ½ teaspoon of butter onto one side of 2 slices of bread. Each sandwich will have 1 slice of bread with butter and 1 slice without.
2. Assemble each sandwich by layering 2 slices of ham, 2 slices of cheese, and 2 slices of tomato on the unbuttered pieces of bread. Top with the other bread slices, buttered side up.
3. Place the sandwiches in the air fryer buttered-side down. Cook for 4 minutes
4. Open the air fryer. Flip the grilled cheese sandwiches. Cook for an additional 4 minutes
5. Cool before serving. Cut each sandwich in half and enjoy.

Cal 525 | Fat 25g | Carb 34g | Protein 41g

## Breakfast Scramble Casserole

**Preparation Time:** 20 minutes | **Cooking Time:** 10 minutes | **Serves:** 4

**Ingredients:**

- 6 slices bacon
- 6 eggs
- Salt
- Pepper
- Cooking oil
- ½ cup chopped red bell pepper
- ½ cup chopped green bell pepper
- ½ cup chopped onion

- ¾ cup shredded Cheddar cheese

**Directions:**

1. In a pan, over medium-high heat, cook the bacon, 5 to 7 minutes, flipping to evenly crisp. Dry out on paper towels, crumble, and set aside. In a medium bowl, whisk the eggs. Add salt and pepper to taste.
2. Spray a barrel pan with cooking oil. Make sure to cover the bottom and sides of the pan. Add the beaten eggs, crumbled bacon, red bell pepper, green bell pepper, and onion to the pan. Place the pan in the air fryer. Cook for 6 minutes Open the air fryer and sprinkle the cheese over the casserole. Cook for an additional 2 minutes. Cool before serving.

Cal 348 | Fat 26g | Carb 4g | Protein 25g

# Spinach Frittata

**Preparation Time:** 5 minutes | **Cooking Time:** 8 minutes | **Serves:** 1

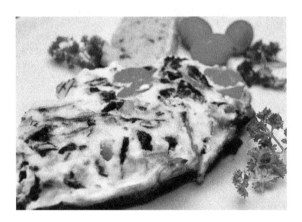

**Ingredients:**

- 3 eggs
- 1 cup spinach, chopped
- 1 small onion, minced
- 2 tbsp mozzarella cheese, grated
- Pepper
- Salt

**Directions:**

1. Preheat the air fryer to 350°F. Spray air fryer pan with cooking spray.
2. In a bowl, whisk eggs with remaining ingredients until well combined.
3. Pour egg mixture into the prepared pan and place pan in the air fryer.

4. Cook frittata for 8 minutes or until set. Serve and enjoy.

Cal 384 | Fat 23g | Carb 11g | Protein 34g

# Classic Hash Browns

**Preparation Time:** 15 minutes | **Cooking Time:** 20 minutes | **Serves:** 4

**Ingredients:**
- 4 russet potatoes
- 1 teaspoon paprika
- Salt
- Pepper
- Cooking oil

**Directions:**
1. Peel the potatoes using a vegetable peeler. Using a cheese grater shred the potatoes. If your grater has different-size holes, use the area of the tool with the largest holes.
2. Put the shredded potatoes in a large bowl of cold water. Let sit for 5 minutes Cold water helps remove excess starch from the potatoes. Stir to help dissolve the starch.
3. Dry out the potatoes and dry with paper towels or napkins. Make sure the potatoes are completely dry.
4. Season the potatoes with the paprika and salt and pepper to taste.
5. Spray the potatoes with cooking oil and transfer them to your Kalorik Maxx Air Fryer. Cook for 20 minutes and shake the basket every 5 minutes (a total of 4 times).
6. Cool before serving.

Cal 150 | Carb 34g | Fiber 5g | Protein 4g

# Canadian Bacon and Cheese Muffins

**Preparation Time:** 5 minutes | **Cooking Time:** 10 minutes | **Serves:** 4

**Ingredients:**
- 4 English muffins
- 8 slices Canadian bacon
- 4 slices cheese
- Cooking oil

**Directions:**

1. Split each English muffin. Assemble the breakfast sandwiches by layering 2 slices of Canadian bacon and 1 slice of cheese onto each English muffin bottom. Put the other half on top of the English muffin. Place the sandwiches in the air fryer. Spray the top of each with cooking oil. Cook for 4 minutes
2. Open the air fryer and flip the sandwiches. Cook for an additional 4 minutes
3. Cool before serving.

Cal 333 | Fat 14g | Carb 27g | Protein 24g

## Radish Hash Browns

**Preparation Time:** 10 minutes | **Cooking Time:** 13 minutes | **Serves:** 4

**Ingredients:**

- 1 lb. radishes, washed and cut off roots
- 1 tbsp olive oil
- 1/2 tsp paprika
- 1/2 tsp onion powder
- 1/2 tsp garlic powder
- 1 medium onion
- 1/4 tsp pepper
- 3/4 tsp sea salt

**Directions:**

1. Slice onion and radishes using a mandolin slicer.
2. Add sliced onion and radishes in a large mixing bowl and toss with olive oil.
3. Transfer onion and radish slices in air fryer and cook at 360°F for 8 minutes Shake basket twice.
4. Return onion and radish slices in a mixing bowl and toss with seasonings.
5. Again, cook onion and radish slices in air fryer for 5 minutes at 400°F. Shake the basket halfway through.
6. Serve and enjoy.

Cal 62 | Fat 3.7g | Carb 7.1g | Protein 1.2g

## Vegetable Egg Cups

**Preparation Time:** 10 minutes | **Cooking Time:** 20 minutes | **Serves:** 4

**Ingredients:**

- 4 eggs
- 1 tbsp cilantro, chopped
- 4 tbsp half and half

- 1 cup cheddar cheese, shredded
- 1 cup vegetables, diced
- Pepper
- Salt

**Directions:**
1. Sprinkle four ramekins with cooking spray and set aside.
2. In a mixing bowl, whisk eggs with cilantro, half and half, vegetables, 1/2 cup cheese, pepper, and salt.
3. Pour egg mixture into the four ramekins.
4. Place ramekins in air fryer and cook at 300°F for 12 minutes
5. Top with remaining 1/2 cup cheese and cook for 2 minutes more at 400°F.
6. Serve and enjoy.

Cal 194 | Fat 11.5g | Carb 6g | Protein 13g

## Omelet Frittata

**Preparation Time:** 10 minutes | **Cooking Time:** 6 minutes | **Serves:** 2

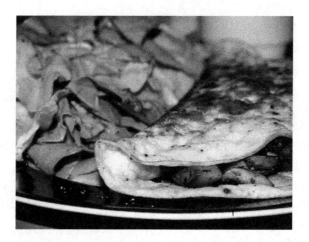

**Ingredients:**
- 3 eggs, lightly beaten
- 2 tbsp cheddar cheese, shredded
- 2 tbsp heavy cream
- 2 mushrooms, sliced
- 1/4 small onion, chopped
- 1/4 bell pepper, diced
- Pepper
- Salt

**Directions:**

1. In a bowl, whisk eggs with cream, vegetables, pepper, and salt.
2. Preheat the air fryer to 400°F.
3. Pour egg mixture into the Kalorik Maxx Air Fryer pan. Place pan in air fryer and cook for 5 minutes
4. Add shredded cheese on top of the frittata and cook for 1 minute more.
5. Serve and enjoy.

Cal 160 | Fat 10g | Carb 4g | Protein 12 g

## Cheese Soufflés

**Preparation Time:** 10 minutes | **Cooking Time:** 6 minutes | **Serves:** 8

**Ingredients:**

- 6 large eggs, separated
- 3/4 cup heavy cream
- 1/4 tsp cayenne pepper
- 1/2 tsp xanthan gum
- 1/2 tsp pepper
- 1/4 tsp cream of tartar
- 2 tbsp chives, chopped
- 2 cups cheddar cheese, shredded
- 1 tsp salt

**Directions:**

1. Preheat the air fryer to 325°F.
2. Spray eight ramekins with cooking spray. Set aside.
3. In a bowl, whisk together almond flour, cayenne pepper, pepper, salt, and xanthan gum.
4. Slowly add heavy cream and mix to combine.
5. Whisk in egg yolks, chives, and cheese until well combined.
6. In a large bowl, add egg whites and cream of tartar and beat until stiff peaks form.
7. Fold egg white mixture into the almond flour mixture until combined.
8. Pour mixture into the prepared ramekins. Divide ramekins in batches.
9. Place the first batch of ramekins into your Kalorik Maxx Air Fryer.
10. Cook soufflé for 20 minutes
11. Serve and enjoy.

Cal 210 | Fat 16g | Carb 1g | Protein 12 g

# Cheese and Red Pepper Egg Cups

**Preparation Time:** 10 minutes | **Cooking Time:** 15 minutes | **Serves:** 4

**Ingredients:**
- Large free-range eggs, 4.
- Shredded cheese, 1 cup
- Diced red pepper, 1 cup
- Half and half, 4 tbsps.
- Salt and Pepper.

**Directions:**
1. Preheat your air fryer to 300°F and grease four ramekins.
2. Grab a medium bowl and add the eggs. Whisk well.
3. Add the red pepper, half the cheese, half and half, and salt and pepper. Stir well to combine.
4. Pour the mixture between the ramekins and pop into your Kalorik Maxx Air Fryer.
5. Cook for 15 minutes then serve and enjoy.

Cal 195 | Fat 12g | Carb 7g | Protein 13g

# Coconut Porridge with Flax Seed

**Preparation Time:** 5 minutes | **Cooking Time:** 30 minutes | **Serves:** 3

**Ingredients:**
- Unsweetened almond milk, 1 ½ cup
- Coconut flour, 2 tbsp.
- Vegan vanilla protein powder, 2 tbsp.
- Powdered erythritol, ¼ tsp.
- Golden flaxseed meal, 3 tbsp.

**Directions:**
1. Preheat your Air Fryer at a temperature of about 375°F
2. Combine coconut flour with the golden flaxseed meal and the protein powder in a bowl
3. Spray your Air Fryer with cooking spray, then pour the mixture in the air fryer pan
4. Pour the milk and top with chopped blueberries and chopped raspberries
5. Move the pan in the air fryer and seal the lid
6. Set the temperature at about 375°F and the timer to about 30 minutes

7. When the timer beeps, turn off your Air Fryer and remove the baking pan
8. Serve and enjoy your delicious porridge!

Cal 249 | Fats: 14g | Carb 6g | Protein 17g

## Easy Chocolate Doughnut

**Preparation Time:** 10 minutes | **Cooking Time:** 12 minutes | **Serves:** 6

**Ingredients:**
- Melted unsalted butter, 3 tbsps.
- Powdered sugar, ¼ cup
- Refrigerated biscuits, 8.
- Semisweet chocolate chips, 48

**Directions:**
1. Cut the biscuits into thirds then flatten them and place 2 chocolate chips at the center.
2. Wrap the chocolate with dough to seal the edges.
3. Rub each dough hole with some butter.
4. Set the dough into your Kalorik Maxx Air Fryer to cook for 12 minutes at 340°F.
5. Set aside to add powdered sugar.
6. Serve and enjoy.

Cal 393 | Fat 17g | Carb 55g | Protein 5g

## Cheesy Spinach Omelet

**Preparation Time:** 5 minutes | **Cooking Time:** 10 minutes | **Serves:** 2

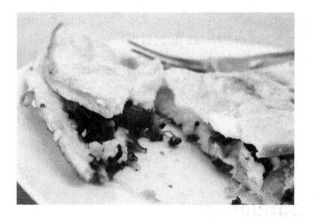

**Ingredients:**

- Eggs, 3
- Chopped fresh spinach, 2 tbsps.
- Shredded cheese, ½ cup
- Pepper.
- Salt.

**Directions:**

1. Mix the eggs with pepper and salt then whisk and put in an oven-safe tray.
2. Add spinach and cheese but do not stir.
3. Allow to cook in the air fryer for 8 minutes at 390°F.
4. Cook for 2 more minutes to brown the omelet.
5. Serve on plates to enjoy.

Cal 209 | Fat 15.9g | Carb 1g | Protein 15.4g

# Roasted Garlic and Thyme Dipping Sauce

**Preparation Time:** 5 minutes | **Cooking Time:** 30 minutes | **Serves:** 1

**Ingredients:**

- Minced fresh thyme leaves, ½ tsp.
- Salt, 1/8 tsp.
- Light mayonnaise, ½ cup
- Crushed roasted garlic, 2 tbsps.
- Pepper, 1/8 tsp.

**Directions:**

1. Wrap garlic in foil. Put it in the cooking basket of the Air Fryer and roast for 30 minutes at 390°F.
2. Combine all the ingredients to serve.

Cal 485 | Fat 39.4g | Carb 34.1g | Protein 2.2g

## Cheesy Sausage and Egg Rolls

**Preparation Time:** 15 minutes | **Cooking Time:** 15 minutes | **Serves:** 8

**Ingredients:**

- Cooked breakfast sausage links, 8 pieces.
- Eggs, 3.
- Salt and Pepper,
- Cheddar cheese slices, 4.
- Refrigerated crescent rolls, 8 oz.

**Directions:**

1. Preheat the air fryer to 325°F.
2. Beat the eggs; reserve one tablespoon as egg wash and scramble the rest.
3. Halve the cheese slices.
4. Separate the dough into 8 triangles.
5. Fill each triangle with a half-slice of cheese, a tablespoon of scrambled eggs, and a sausage link.
6. Loosely roll up all filled triangles before placing in the air fryer. Brush with the egg wash that was set aside and sprinkle all over with pepper and salt.
7. Cook for 15 minutes.
8. Serve right away.

Cal 270 | Fat 20.0g | Protein 10.0g | Carb 13.0 g

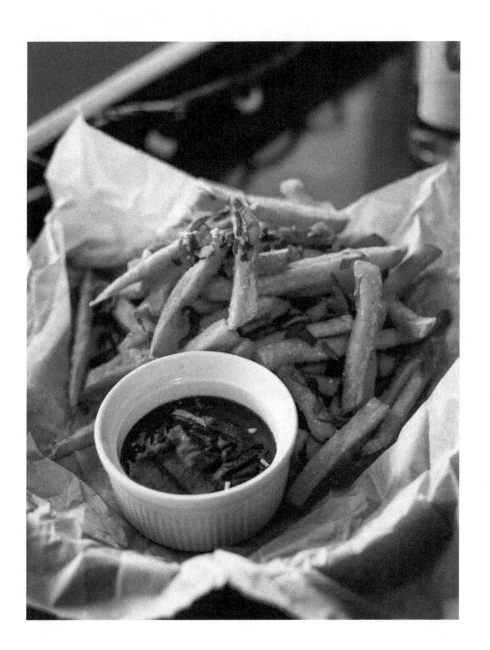

# Snacks & Appetizers

## Balsamic Zucchini Slices

**Preparation Time:** 5 minutes | **Cooking Time:** 50 minutes | **Serves:** 6

**Ingredients:**
- zucchinis, thinly sliced
- Salt and black pepper to taste
- tablespoons avocado oil
- tablespoons balsamic vinegar

**Directions:**
1. Put all of the ingredients into a bowl and mix.
2. Put the zucchini mixture in your air fryer's basket and cook at 220°F for 50 minutes.
3. Serve as a snack and enjoy!

Cal 40 | Fat 3g | Fiber 7g | Carb 3g | Protein 7g

## Burrata-Stuffed Tomatoes

**Preparation Time:** 5 minutes | **Cooking Time:** 5 minutes | **Serves:** 4

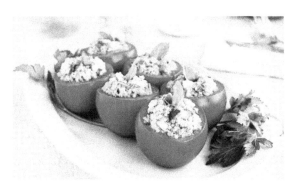

**Ingredients:**

- 4 medium tomatoes
- ½ teaspoon fine sea salt
- 4 (2-ounce) Burrata balls
- Fresh basil leaves, for garnish
- Extra-virgin olive oil, for drizzling

**Directions**

1. Preparing the Ingredients. Preheat the air fryer to 300°F.
2. Scoop out the tomato seeds and membranes using a melon baller or spoon. Sprinkle the insides of the tomatoes with the salt. Stuff each tomato with a ball of Burrata.
3. Air Frying. Put it in the fryer and cook for 5 minutes, or until the cheese has softened.
4. Garnish with olive oil and basil leaves. Serve warm.

Cal 108 | Fat 7g | Protein 6g | Carb 5g | Fiber 2g

## Turmeric Carrot Chips

**Preparation Time:** 5 minutes | **Cooking Time:** 25 minutes | **Serves:** 4

**Ingredients:**

- carrots, thinly sliced
- Salt and black pepper to taste
- ½ teaspoon turmeric powder
- ½ teaspoon chaat masala
- 1 teaspoon olive oil

**Directions:**

1. Put all of the ingredients in a bowl and toss well.
2. Put the mixture in your air fryer's basket and cook at 370°F for 25 minutes, shaking the fryer from time to time.
3. Serve as a snack.

Cal 161 | Fat 1g | Fiber 2g | Carb 5g | Protein 3g

## Pesto Tomatoes

**Preparation Time:** 5 minutes | **Cooking Time:** 10 minutes | **Serves:** 4

**Ingredients:**

- Large heirloom tomatoes – 3, cut into ½ inch thick slices.
- Pesto – 1 cup
- Feta cheese – 8 oz. cut into ½ inch thick slices
- Red onion – ½ cup, sliced thinly

- Olive oil – 1 tbsp.

**Directions:**
1. Spread some pesto on each slice of tomato. Top each tomato slice with a feta slice and onion and drizzle with oil. Arrange the tomatoes onto the greased rack and spray with cooking spray.
2. Preheat the Air Fryer to 390°F.
3. Arrange the drip pan in the bottom of Air Fryer Oven cooking chamber and cook for 14 minutes.
4. Serve warm.

Cal 480 | Carb 13g | Fat 41.9g | Protein 15.4g

# Crisp Kale

**Preparation Time:** 5 Minutes | **Cooking Time:** 8 Minutes | **Serves:** 2

**Ingredients:**
- 4 Handfuls Kale, Washed & Stemless
- 1 Tablespoon Olive Oil
- Pinch Sea Salt

**Directions:**
1. Start by heating it to 360°F, and then combine your ingredients together making sure your kale is coated evenly.
2. Place the kale in your fryer and cook for 8 minutes.

Cal 121 | Fat 4g | Carb 5g | Protein 8g

# Chives Radish Snack

**Preparation Time:** 5 minutes | **Cooking Time:** 10 minutes | **Serves:** 4

**Ingredients:**
- 16 radishes, sliced
- A drizzle of olive oil
- Salt and black pepper to taste
- 1 tablespoon chives, chopped

**Directions:**
1. In a bowl, mix the radishes, salt, pepper, and oil; toss well.
2. Place the radishes in your air fryer's basket and cook at 350°F for 10 minutes.
3. Divide into bowls and serve with chives sprinkled on top.

Cal 100 | Fat 1g | Fiber 2g | Carb 4g | Protein 1g

# Lentils Snack

**Preparation Time:** 5 Minutes | **Cooking Time:** 12 minutes | **Serves:** 4

**Ingredients:**

- 15 ounces canned lentils, drained
- ½ teaspoon cumin, ground
- 1 tablespoon olive oil
- 1 teaspoon sweet paprika
- Salt and black pepper to taste

**Directions:**

1. Place all ingredients in a bowl and blend it well.
2. Transfer the mixture to your air fryer and cook at 400°F for 12 minutes.
3. Divide into bowls and serve as a snack or a side, or appetizer!

Cal 151 | Fat 1g | Fiber 6g | Carb 10g | Protein 6g

---

# Jicama Fries

**Preparation Time:** 10 minutes | **Cooking Time:** 5 minutes | **Serves:** 4

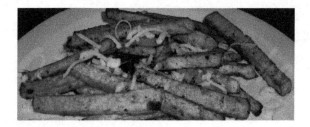

**Ingredients:**

- 1 tbsp. dried thyme
- ¾ C. arrowroot flour
- ½ large Jicama
- eggs

**Directions:**

1. Preparing the Ingredients. Sliced jicama into fries.
2. Whisk eggs together and pour over fries. Toss to coat.
3. Mix a pinch of salt, thyme, and arrowroot flour together. Toss egg-coated jicama into dry mixture, tossing to coat well.
4. Air Frying. Spray the air fryer basket with olive oil and add fries. Set temperature to 350°F, and set time to 5 minutes. Toss halfway into the cooking process.

Cal 211 | Fat 19g | Carbs 16g | Protein 9g

# Air Fried Corn

**Preparation Time:** 5 minutes | **Cooking Time:** 10 minutes | **Serves:** 4

**Ingredients:**
- tablespoons corn kernels
- 2½ tablespoons butter

**Directions:**
1. In a saucepan that fits your air fryer, mix the corn with the butter.
2. Place the pan inside the air fryer and cook at 400°F for 10 minutes.
3. Serve as a snack and enjoy!

Cal 70 | Fat 2g | Fiber 2g | Carb 7g | Protein 3g

# Tuna Zucchini Melts

**Preparation Time**: 15 minutes | **Cooking Time**: 5 minutes | **Serves**: 4

**Ingredients**:
- corn tortillas
- tablespoons softened butter
- 1 (6-ounce) can chunk light tuna, drained
- 1 cup shredded zucchini, drained by squeezing in a kitchen towel
- ⅓ cup mayonnaise
- tablespoons mustard
- 1 cup shredded Cheddar or Colby cheese

**Directions**:
1. Spread the tortillas with the softened butter. Place in the air fryer basket and grill for 2 to 3 minutes or until the tortillas are crisp. Remove from basket and set aside.
2. In a medium bowl, combine the tuna, zucchini, mayonnaise, and mustard, and mix well.
3. Divide the tuna mixture among the toasted tortillas. Top each with some of the shredded cheese.
4. Grill in the air fryer for 2 to 4 minutes or until the tuna mixture is hot, and the cheese melts and starts to brown. Serve.

Cal 428 | Fat 30g | Carb 19g | Fiber 3g | Protein 22g

# Breaded Mushrooms

**Preparation Time:** 10 minutes | **Cooking Time:** 45 minutes | **Serves:** 4

**Ingredients:**

- 1 lb. small Button mushrooms, cleaned
- cups breadcrumbs
- eggs, beaten
- Salt and pepper to taste
- 2 cups Parmigiano Reggiano cheese, grated

**Directions:**
1. Preheat the Air Fryer to 360°F. Pour the breadcrumbs in a bowl, add salt and pepper and mix well. Pour the cheese in a separate bowl and set aside. Dip each mushroom in the eggs, then in the crumbs, and then in the cheese.
2. Slide out the fryer basket and add 6 to 10 mushrooms. Cook them for 20 minutes, in batches, if needed. Serve with cheese dip.

Cal 487 | Carb 49g | Fat 22g | Protein 31g

---

# Hot Chicken Wingettes

**Preparation Time:** 10 minutes | **Cooking Time:** 40 minutes | **Serves:** 4

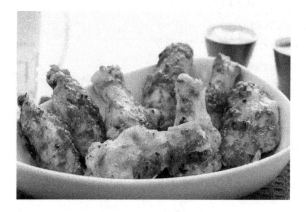

**Ingredients:**
- 15 chicken wingettes
- Salt and pepper to taste
- ⅓ cup hot sauce
- ⅓ cup butter
- ½ tbsp vinegar

**Directions**
1. Preheat the Air Fryer to 360°F. Season the vignettes with pepper and salt.

2. Add them to your Kalorik Maxx Air Fryer and cook for 35 minutes. Toss every 5 minutes. Once ready, remove them into a bowl. Over low heat melt the butter in a saucepan.
3. Add the vinegar and hot sauce. Stir and cook for a minute.
4. Turn the heat off. Pour the sauce over the chicken. Toss to coat well. Transfer the chicken to a serving platter.
5. Serve with blue cheese dressing.

Cal 563 | Carb 2g | Fat 28g | Protein 35g

# Cheesy Sticks with Sweet Thai Sauce

**Preparation Time:** 2 hours | **Cooking Time:** 20 minutes | **Serves:** 4

**Ingredients:**
- 12 mozzarella string cheese
- cups breadcrumbs
- eggs
- 1 cup sweet Thai sauce
- tbsp skimmed milk

**Directions**
1. Pour the crumbs in a medium bowl. Break the eggs into a different bowl and beat with the milk. One after the other, dip each cheese sticks in the egg mixture, in the crumbs, then egg mixture again and then in the crumbs again.
2. Place the coated cheese sticks on a cookie sheet and freeze for 1 to 2 hours. Preheat the Air Fryer to 380°F.
3. Arrange the sticks in the fryer without overcrowding. Cook for 5 minutes, flipping them halfway through cooking to brown evenly. Cook in batches.
4. Serve with a sweet Thai sauce.

Cal 158 | Carb 14g | Fat 7g | Protein 9g

# Bacon Wrapped Avocados

**Preparation Time:** 10 minutes | **Cooking Time:** 30 minutes | **Serves:** 4

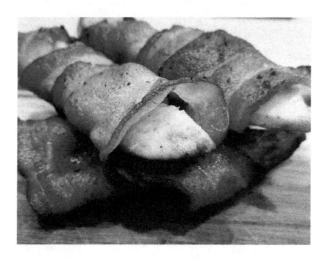

**Ingredients:**

- 12 thick strips bacon
- large avocados, sliced
- ⅓ tsp salt
- ⅓ tsp chili powder
- ⅓ tsp cumin powder

**Directions**

1. Stretch the bacon strips to elongate and use a knife to cut in half to make 24 pieces. Wrap each bacon piece around a slice of avocado from one end to the other end. Tuck the end of bacon into the wrap. Arrange on a flat surface and season with salt, chili and cumin on both sides.
2. Arrange 4 to 8 wrapped pieces in the air fryer and cook at 350°F for 8 minutes, or until the bacon is browned and crunchy, flipping halfway through to cook evenly. Remove onto a wire rack and repeat the process for the remaining avocado pieces.

Cal 193 | Carb 10g | Fat 16g | Protein 4g

# Crispy Brussels Sprouts

**Preparation Time:** 5 minutes | **Cooking Time:** 10 minutes | **Serves:** 2

**Ingredients:**

- ½ pound brussels sprouts, cut in half
- ½ tablespoon oil
- ½ tablespoon unsalted butter, melted

**Directions:**

1. Rub sprouts with oil and place into your Kalorik Maxx Air Fryer basket.

2. Cook at 400°F for 10 minutes. Stir once at the halfway mark.
3. Remove the air fryer basket and drizzle with melted butter.
4. Serve.

Cal 90 | Fat 6.1g | Carb 4g | Protein 2.9g

## Carrot Crisps

**Preparation Time:** 10 minutes | **Cooking Time:** 10 minutes | **Serves:** 4

**Ingredients:**
- large carrots, washed and peeled
- Salt to taste
- Cooking spray

**Directions**
1. Using a mandolin slicer, slice the carrots very thinly height wise. Put the carrot strips in a bowl and season with salt to taste. Grease the fryer basket lightly with cooking spray, and add the carrot strips.
2. Cook at 350°F for 10 minutes, stirring once halfway through.

Cal 35 | Carb 8g | Fat 3g | Protein 1g

## Garlicky Bok Choy

**Preparation Time:** 10 minutes | **Cooking Time:** 10 minutes | **Serves:** 2

**Ingredients:**
- bunches baby bok choy
- spray oil
- 1 tsp garlic powder

**Directions:**
1. Toss bok choy with garlic powder and spread them in the Air fryer. Spray them with cooking oil.
2. Select the Air Fry mode at 350°F temperature for 6 minutes.
3. Serve fresh.

Cal 81 | Protein 0.4g | Carb 4.7g | Fat 8.3g

## Bacon-Wrapped Asparagus

**Preparation Time:** 5 minutes | **Cooking Time:** 10 minutes | **Serves:** 4

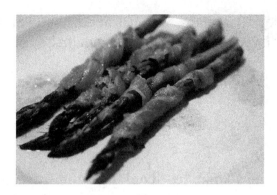

**Ingredients:**
- 1 pound asparagus, trimmed (about 24 spears)
- 4slices bacon or beef bacon
- ½ cup Ranch Dressin for serving
- 3 tablespoons chopped fresh chives, for garnish

**Directions**
1. Preparing the Ingredients. Grease the air fryer basket with avocado oil. Preheat the air fryer to 400°F.
2. Slice the bacon down the middle, making long, thin strips. Wrap 1 slice of bacon around 3 asparagus spears and secure each end with a toothpick. Repeat with the remaining bacon and asparagus.
3. Air Frying. Place the asparagus bundles in the air fryer in a single layer.
4. Cook for 8 minutes for thin stalks, 10 minutes for medium to thick stalks, or until the asparagus is slightly charred on the ends and the bacon is crispy.
5. Serve with ranch dressing and garnish with chives. Best served fresh.

Cal 241 | Fat 22g | Protein 7g | Carb 6g | Fiber 3g

## Quick Cheese Sticks

**Preparation Time:** 5 minutes | **Cooking Time:** 10 minutes | **Serves:** 4

**Ingredients:**
- 6 oz bread cheese
- tbsp butter
- cups panko crumbs

**Directions**
1. Place the butter in a dish and melt it in the microwave, for 2 minutes; set aside. With a knife, cut the cheese into equal sized sticks.
2. Brush each stick with butter and dip into panko crumbs. Arrange the cheese sticks in a single layer on the fryer basket.

3. Cook at 390°F for 10 minutes. Flip them halfway through, to brown evenly; serve warm.

Cal 256 | Carb 8g | Fat 21g | Protein 16g

# Radish Chips

**Preparation Time:** 10 minutes | **Cooking Time:** 20 minutes | **Serves:** 4

**Ingredients:**
- radishes, leaves removed and cleaned
- Salt to season
- Water
- Cooking spray

**Directions**
1. Using a mandolin, slice the radishes thinly. Put them in a pot and pour water on them. Heat the pot on a stovetop, and bring to boil, until the radishes are translucent, for 4 minutes. After 4 minutes, drain the radishes through a sieve; set aside. Grease the fryer basket with cooking spray.
2. Add in the radish slices and cook for 8 minutes, flipping once halfway through. Cook until golden brown, at 400°F. Meanwhile, prepare a paper towel-lined plate. Once the radishes are ready, transfer them to the paper towel-lined plate. Season with salt, and serve with ketchup or garlic mayo.

Cal 25 | Carb 0.2g | Fat 2g | Protein 0.1g

# Herbed Croutons with Brie Cheese

**Preparation Time:** 10 minutes | **Cooking Time:** 10 minutes | **Serves:** 4

**Ingredients:**
- tbsp olive oil
- 1 tbsp french herbs
- oz brie cheese, chopped
- slices bread, halved

**Directions**
1. Warm up your Air Fryer to 340° F.
2. Using a bowl, mix oil with herbs.
3. Dip the bread slices in the oil mixture to coat.
4. Place the coated slices on a flat surface. Lay the brie cheese on the slices.
5. Place the slices into your air fryer's basket and cook for 7 minutes.
6. Once the bread is ready, cut into cubes.

Cal 20 | Carb 1.5g | Fat 1.3g | Protein 0.5g

# Chia Seed Crackers

**Preparation Time:** 15 minutes | **Cooking Time:** 45 minutes | **Serves:** 48

**Ingredients:**
- 1 Cup raw chia seed
- 3/4 Teaspoon salt
- 1/4 Teaspoon garlic powder
- 1/4 Teaspoon onion powder
- 1 Cup cold water

**Directions:**
1. Put the chia seeds in a bowl. Add salt, garlic powder, and onion powder.
2. Pour into the water. Stir. Cover with plastic wrap. Store in the fridge overnight.
3. Preheat the Air fryer toaster oven to 200°F. Cover a baking sheet with a silicone mat or parchment.
4. Transfer the soaked linseed to a prepared baking sheet. Scatter it out with a spatula in a thin, flat rectangle about 1 cm thick. Rate the rectangle in about 32 small rectangles.
5. Bake in the preheated Air fryer toaster oven up to the chia seeds have darkened and contract slightly, about 3 hours. Let it cool. Break individual cookies.

Cal 120 | Fat 3.9g | Carb 1.9g | Protein 1.9g

# Stuffed Jalapeno

**Preparation Time:** 10 minutes | **Cooking Time:** 10 minutes | **Serves:** 4

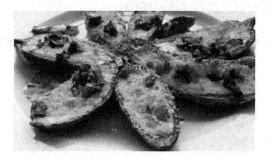

**Ingredients:**
- 1 lb. ground pork sausage
- 1 (8 oz.) package cream cheese, softened
- 1 cup shredded Parmesan cheese
- 1 lb. large fresh jalapeno peppers halved lengthwise and seeded
- 1 (8 oz.) bottle Ranch dressing

**Directions:**

1. in Mix pork sausage ground with ranch dressing and cream cheese in a bowl. But the jalapeno in half and remove their seeds. Divide the cream cheese mixture into the jalapeno halves.
2. Place the jalapeno pepper in a baking tray. Set the Baking tray inside the Air Fryer toaster oven and close the lid. Select the Bake mode at 350°F for 10 minutes. Serve warm.

Cal 168| Protein 9.4g | Carb 12.1g | Fat 21.2g

## Flax Seed Chips

**Preparation Time:** 5 minutes | **Cooking Time:** 15 minutes | **Serves:** 4

**Ingredients:**

- 1 Cup almond flour
- 1/2 Cup flax seeds
- 1 1/2 Teaspoons seasoned salt
- 1 Teaspoon sea salt
- 1/2 Cup water

**Directions:**

1. Preheat the Air fryer toaster oven to 340°F.
2. Combine almond flour, flax seeds, 1 1/2 teaspoons seasoned salt and sea salt in a container; Stir in the water up to the dough is completely mixed.
3. Shape the dough into narrow size slices the size of a bite and place them on a baking sheet. Sprinkle the rounds with seasoned salt.
4. Bake in preheated air fryer toaster oven up to crispy, about 15 minutes.
5. Cool fully and store in an airtight box or in a sealed bag.

Cal 126.9 | Fat 6.1g | Carb 15.9g | Protein 2.9g

## Salted Hazelnuts

**Preparation Time:** 15 minutes | **Cooking Time:** 10 minutes | **Serves:** 8

**Ingredients:**

- Cups dry roasted Hazelnuts, no salt added
- Tablespoons coconut oil
- 1 Teaspoon garlic powder
- 1 Sprig fresh Thyme, chopped
- 1 1/2 Teaspoons salt

**Directions:**

1. Preheat the Air fryer toaster oven to 350°F.

2. Mix the Hazelnuts, coconut oil, garlic powder and thyme in a bowl until the nuts are fully covered. Sprinkle with salt. Spread evenly on a baking sheet.
3. Bake in the preheated Air fryer toaster oven for 10 minutes.

Cal 237 | Fat 21.3g | Carb 5.9g | Protein 7.4g

## Cajun Olives and Peppers

**Preparation Time:** 4 minutes | **Cooking Time:** 12 minutes | **Serves:** 4

**Ingredients:**
- 1 tablespoon olive oil
- ½ pound mixed bell peppers, sliced
- 1 cup black olives, pitted and halved
- ½ tablespoon Cajun seasoning

**Directions:**
1. In a pan that fits the air fryer, combine all the ingredients.
2. Put the pan it in your air fryer and cook at 390°F for 12 minutes.
3. Divide the mix between plates and serve.

Cal 151 | Fat 3g | Fiber 2g | Carb 4g | Protein 5g

## Green Beans & Bacon

**Preparation Time:** 15 minutes | **Cooking Time:** 20 minutes | **Serves:** 4

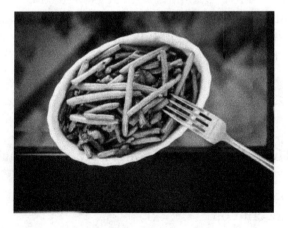

**Ingredients:**
- 3 cups frozen cut green beans
- 1 medium onion, chopped
- 3slices bacon, chopped

- ¼ cup water
- Kosher salt and black pepper

**Directions:**

1. Preparing the Ingredients
2. In a 6 × 3-inch round heatproof pan, combine the frozen green beans, onion, bacon, and water. Toss to combine. Place the saucepan in the basket.
3. Air Frying . Set the air fryer to 375°F for 15 minutes.
4. Raise the air fryer temperature to 400°F for 5 minutes. Season the beans with salt and pepper to taste and toss well.
5. Remove the pan from the air fryer basket and cover with foil. Let it rest for 5 minutes then serve.

Cal 230 | Fat 10g | Carb 14g | Protein 17g

## Wrapped Asparagus

**Preparation Time:** 10 minutes | **Cooking Time:** 5 minutes | **Serves:** 4

**Ingredients:**

- 12 ounces asparagus
- ½ teaspoon ground black pepper
- 3-ounce turkey fillet, sliced
- ¼ teaspoon chili flakes

**Directions:**

1. Sprinkle the asparagus with the ground black pepper and chili flakes.
2. Stir carefully.
3. Wrap the asparagus in the sliced turkey fillet and place in the air fryer basket.
4. Cook the asparagus at 400° F for 5 minutes, turning halfway through cooking.
5. Let the wrapped asparagus cool for 2 minutes before serving.

Cal 133 | Fat 9g | Fiber 1.9g | Carbs 3.8g | Protein 9.8g

## Yogurt Bread

**Preparation Time:** 20 minutes | **Cooking Time:** 40 minutes | **Serves:** 10

**Ingredients:**

- 1½ cups warm water, divided
- 1½ teaspoons active dry yeast
- 1 teaspoon sugar
- 3 cups all-purpose flour
- 1 cup plain Greek yogurt
- 2 teaspoons kosher salt

**Directions:**

1. Add ½ cup of the warm water, yeast and sugar in the bowl of a stand mixer, fitted with the dough hook attachment and mix well.
2. Set aside for about 5 minutes
3. Add the flour, yogurt, and salt and mix on medium-low speed until the dough comes together.
4. Then, mix on medium speed for 5 minutes
5. Place the dough into a bowl.
6. With a plastic wrap, cover the bowl and place in a warm place for about 2-3 hours or until doubled in size.
7. Transfer the dough onto a lightly floured surface and shape into a smooth ball.
8. Place the dough onto a greased parchment paper-lined rack.
9. With a kitchen towel, cover the dough and let rest for 15 minutes
10. With a very sharp knife, cut a 4x½-inch deep cut down the center of the dough.
11. Take to the preheated air fryer at 325°F for 40 minutes.
12. Carefully, invert the bread to cool completely before slicing.
13. Cut the bread into desired-sized slices and serve.

Cal 157 | Fat 0.7g | Carb 31g | Protein 5.5g

## Fried Plantains

**Preparation Time:** 5 minutes | **Cooking Time:** 10 minutes | **Serves:** 2

**Ingredients:**

- 2ripe plantains, peeled and cut at a diagonal into ½-inch-thick pieces
- 3 tablespoons ghee, melted
- ¼ teaspoon kosher salt

**Directions**

1. Preparing the Ingredients. In a bowl, mix the plantains with the ghee and salt.
2. Air Frying. Arrange the plantain pieces in the air fryer basket. Set the air fryer to 400°F for 8 minutes. The plantains are done when they are soft and tender on the inside, and have plenty of crisp, sweet, brown spots on the outside.

Cal 180 | Fat 5g | Carb 10g | Protein 7g

## Chili Corn on the Cob

**Preparation Time:** 10 minutes | **Cooking Time:** 15 minutes | **Serves:** 4

**Ingredients:**

- 2tablespoon olive oil, divided
- 2 tablespoons grated Parmesan cheese

- 1 teaspoon garlic powder
- 1 teaspoon chili powder
- 1 teaspoon ground cumin
- 1 teaspoon paprika
- 1 teaspoon salt
- ¼ teaspoon cayenne pepper (optional)
- 4ears fresh corn, shucked

**Directions:**
1. Grease the air fryer basket with 1 tablespoon of olive oil. Set aside.
2. Combine the Parmesan cheese, garlic powder, chili powder, cumin, paprika, salt, and cayenne pepper (if desired) in a small bowl and stir to mix well.
3. Lightly coat the ears of corn with the remaining 1 tablespoon of olive oil. Rub the cheese mixture all over the ears of corn until completely coated.
4. Arrange the ears of corn in the greased basket in a single layer.
5. Put in the air fryer basket and cook at 400°F for 15 minutes.
6. Flip the ears of corn halfway through the cooking time.
7. When cooking is complete, they should be lightly browned. Remove from the oven and let them cool for 5 minutes before serving.

Cal 172 | Fat 9.8g |Carb 17.5g | Protein 3.9g

# Allspice Chicken Wings

**Preparation Time:| Cooking Time:** 45 minutes | **Serves:** 8

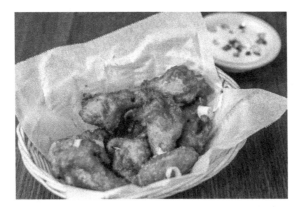

**Ingredients:**
- ½ tsp celery salt
- ½ tsp bay leaf powder
- ½ tsp ground black pepper

- ½ tsp paprika
- ¼ tsp dry mustard
- ¼ tsp cayenne pepper
- ¼ tsp allspice
- 2 pounds chicken wings

**Directions:**
1. Grease the air fryer basket and preheat to 340°F. In a bowl, mix celery salt, bay leaf powder, black pepper, paprika, dry mustard, cayenne pepper, and allspice. Coat the wings thoroughly in this mixture.
2. Arrange the wings in an even layer in the basket of the air fryer. Cook the chicken until it's no longer pinks around the bone, for 30 minutes then, increase the temperature to 380°F and cook for 6 minutes more, until crispy on the outside.

Cal 332 | Fat 10.1g | Carb 31.3g | Protein 12 g

## Simple Stuffed Potatoes

**Preparation Time:** 15 Minutes | **Cooking Time:** 35 Minutes | **Serves:** 4

**Ingredients:**
- 4 Large Potatoes, Peeled
- 2 Bacon, Rashers
- ½ Brown Onion, Diced
- ¼ Cup Cheese, Grated

**Directions:**
1. Start by heating your air fryer to 350°F.
2. Cut your potatoes in half, and then brush the potatoes with oil.
3. Put it in your air fryer, and cook for ten minutes. Brush the potatoes with oil again and bake for another ten minutes.
4. Make a whole in the baked potato to get them ready to stuff.
5. Sauté the bacon and onion in a frying pan. You should do this over medium heat, adding cheese and stir. Remove from heat.
6. Stuff your potatoes, and cook for four to five minutes.

Cal 180 | Fat 8g | Carb 10g | Protein 11g

## Ravishing Carrots with Honey Glaze

**Preparation Time:** 5 minutes | **Cooking Time:** 11 minutes | **Serves:** 1

**Ingredients:**

- 3 cups of chopped into ½-inch pieces carrots
- 1 tablespoon of olive oil
- 2 tablespoons of honey
- 1 tablespoon of brown sugar
- salt and black pepper

**Directions:**
1. Heat up your air fryer to 390°F.
2. Using a bowl, add and toss the carrot pieces, olive oil, honey, brown sugar, salt, and the black pepper until it is properly covered.
3. Place it inside your air fryer and add the seasoned glazed carrots.
4. Cook it for 5 minutes at 390°F, and then shake after 6 minutes. Serve and enjoy!

Cal 90 | Fat 3.5g | Fiber 2g | Carb 13g | Protein 1g

# Sweet Potato Fries

**Preparation Time:** 10 Minutes | **Cooking Time:** 12 Minutes | **Serves:** 2

**Ingredients:**
- 3 Large Sweet Potatoes, Peeled
- 1 Tablespoon Olive Oil
- A Pinch Teaspoon Sea Salt

**Directions:**
1. Turn on your air fryer to 390°F.
2. Start by cutting your sweet potatoes in quarters, cutting them lengthwise to make fries.
3. Combine the uncooked fries with a tablespoon of sea salt and olive oil. Make sure all of your fries are coated well.
4. Place your sweet potato pieces in your air fryer, cooking for 12 minutes.
5. Cook for two to three minutes more if you want it to be crispier.
6. Add more salt to taste, and serve when cooled.

Cal: 150 | Fat: 6g | Carbs: 8g | Protein: 9g

# Meat recipes

## BBQ Pork Ribs

**Preparation Time:** 10 minutes | **Cooking Time:** 12 minutes | **Serves:** 6

**Ingredients:**

- 1 slab baby back pork ribs, cut into pieces
- ½ cup BBQ sauce
- ½ tsp paprika
- Salt

**Directions:**

1. Add pork ribs in a mixing bowl.
2. Add BBQ sauce, paprika, and salt over pork ribs and coat well and set aside for 30 minutes.
3. Preheat the Air Fryer oven to 350°F.
4. Arrange marinated pork ribs on Air Fryer oven pan and cook for 10-12 minutes. Turn halfway through.
5. Serve and enjoy.

Cal 145 | Fat 7g | Carb 10g | Sugar 7g | Protein 9 g

## Greek Lamb Chops

**Preparation Time:** 10 minutes | **Cooking Time:** 10 minutes | **Serves:** 4

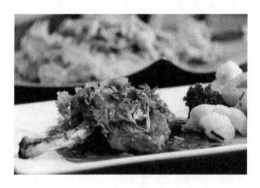

**Ingredients:**

- 2 lbs. lamb chops
- 2 tsp garlic, minced
- 1 ½ tsp dried oregano
- ¼ cup fresh lemon juice
- salt and pepper

**Directions:**
1. Add lamb chops in a mixing bowl. Add remaining ingredients over the lamb chops and coat well.
2. Arrange lamb chops on the air fryer oven tray and cook at 400°F for 5 minutes.
3. Turn lamb chops and cook for 5 minutes more.
4. Serve and enjoy.

Cal 538 | Fat 29.4g | Carb 1.3g | Sugar 0.4g | Protein 64 g

# Easy Rosemary Lamb Chops

**Preparation Time:** 10 minutes | **Cooking Time:** 6 minutes | **Serves:** 4

**Ingredients:**
- 4 lamb chops
- 2 tbsp dried rosemary
- ¼ cup fresh lemon juice
- Pepper
- Salt

**Directions:**
1. In a small bowl, mix together lemon juice, rosemary, pepper, and salt.
2. Brush lemon juice rosemary mixture over lamb chops.
3. Place lamb chops on air fryer oven tray and air fry at 400°F for 3 minutes.
4. Turn lamb chops to the other side and cook for 3 minutes more.
5. Serve and enjoy.

Cal 267 | Fat 21.7g | Carb 1.4g | Sugar 0.3g | Protein 16.9 g

# Juicy Steak Bites

**Preparation Time:** 10 minutes | **Cooking Time:** 9 minutes | **Serves:** 4

**Ingredients:**
- 1 lb sirloin steak, sliced into bite-size pieces
- 1 tbsp steak seasoning
- 1 tbsp olive oil
- Pepper
- Salt

**Directions:**

1. Preheat the air fryer oven to 390°F.
2. Add steak pieces into the large mixing bowl. Add steak seasoning, oil, pepper, and salt over steak pieces and toss until well coated.
3. Transfer steak pieces on Air Fryer pan and air fry for 5 minutes.
4. Turn steak pieces to the other side and cook for 4 minutes more.
5. Serve and enjoy.

Cal 241 | Fat 10.6g | Carb 0g | Sugar 0g | Protein 34.4 g

## Simple Beef Patties

**Preparation Time:** 10 minutes | **Cooking Time:** 13 minutes | **Serves:** 4

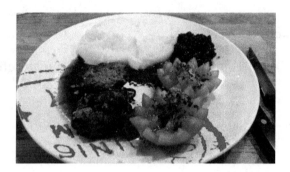

**Ingredients:**

- 1 lb. ground beef
- ½ tsp garlic powder
- ¼ tsp onion powder
- Pepper
- Salt

**Directions:**

1. Preheat the Air Fryer oven to 400°F.
2. Add ground meat, garlic powder, onion powder, pepper, and salt into the mixing bowl and mix until well combined.
3. Make even shape patties from meat mixture and arrange on air fryer pan.
4. Place pan in Air Fryer oven.
5. Cook patties for 10 minutes. Turn patties after 5 minutes.
6. Serve and enjoy.

Cal 212 | Fat 7.1g | Carb 0.4g | Sugar 0.1g | Protein 34.5 g

# Spiced Butternut Squash

**Preparation Time:** 10 minutes **Cooking Time:** 15 minutes | **Serves:** 4

**Ingredients:**

- 4 cups 1-inch-cubed butternut squash
- 2 tablespoons vegetable oil
- 1 to 2 tablespoons brown sugar
- 1 teaspoon Chinese five-spice powder

## Directions

1. Preparing the Ingredients. In a bowl, combine the oil, sugar, squash, and five-spice powder. Toss to coat.
2. Place the squash in the air fryer basket.
3. Air Frying. Set the air fryer to 400°F for 15 minutes or until tender.

Cal 160 | Fat 5g | Carbs 9g | Protein 6g

# Easy Beef Roast

**Preparation Time:** 10 minutes | **Cooking Time:** 45 minutes | **Serves:** 6

**Ingredients:**

- 2 ½ lbs. beef roast
- 2 tbsp Italian seasoning

**Directions:**

1. Arrange roast on the rotisserie spite.
2. Rub roast with Italian seasoning then insert into your Kalorik Maxx Air Fryer oven.
3. Air fry at 350°F for 45 minutes or until the internal temperature of the roast reaches to 145 F.
4. Slice and serve.

Cal 365 | Fat 13.2g | Carb 0.5g | Sugar 0.4g | Protein 57.4 g

# Beef Jerky

**Preparation Time:** 10 minutes | **Cooking Time:** 4 hours | **Serves:** 4

**Ingredients:**

- 2 lbs. London broil, sliced thinly
- 1 tsp onion powder

- 3 tbsp brown sugar
- 3 tbsp soy sauce
- 1 tsp olive oil

**Directions:**
1. Add all ingredients except meat in the large zip-lock bag.
2. Mix until well combined. Add meat in the bag.
3. Seal bag and massage gently to cover the meat with marinade.
4. Let marinate the meat for 1 hour.
5. Arrange marinated meat slices on Air Fryer tray and dehydrate at 160°F for 4 hours.

Cal 133 | Fat 4.7g | Carb 9.4g | Sugar 7.1g | Protein 13.4 g

## Pork Taquitos

**Preparation Time:** 10 minutes | **Cooking Time:** 16 minutes | **Serves:** 8

**Ingredients:**
- 1 juiced lime
- 10 whole wheat tortillas
- 2 ½ c. Shredded mozzarella cheese
- 30 ounces of cooked and shredded pork tenderloin

**Directions:**
1. Preparing the ingredients. Ensure your air fryer is preheated to 380°F.
2. Drizzle pork with lime juice and gently mix.
3. Heat up tortillas in the microwave with a dampened paper towel to soften.
4. Add about 3 ounces of pork and ¼ cup of shredded cheese to each tortilla. Tightly roll them up.
5. Grease the air fryer basket with a drizzle of olive oil.
6. Air frying. Set temperature to 380°F, and set time to 10 minutes. Air fry taquitos 7-10 minutes till tortillas turn a slight golden color, making sure to flip halfway through cooking process.

Cal 309 | Fat 11g | Protein 21g

## Panko-Breaded Pork Chops

**Preparation Time:** 5 minutes | **Cooking Time:** 12 minutes | **Serves:** 6

**Ingredients:**
- 5 (3½- to 5-ounce) pork chops (bone-in or boneless)

- salt and pepper
- ¼ cup all-purpose flour
- 2 tablespoons panko bread crumbs
- Cooking oil

**Directions:**
1. Preparing the Ingredients. Season the pork chops with salt and pepper to taste.
2. Sprinkle the flour on both sides of the pork chops, then coat both sides with panko bread crumbs.
3. Put the pork chops in the air fryer. Stacking them is okay.
4. Air Frying. Spray the pork chops with cooking oil. Cook for 6 minutes.
5. Halfway through, flip the pork chops. Cook for an additional 6 minutes
6. Cool before serving.
7. Typically, bone-in pork chops are juicier than boneless. If you prefer really juicy pork chops, use bone-in.

Cal 246 | Fat 13g | Protein 26g |Fiber 0g

# Crispy Roast Garlic-Salt Pork

**Preparation Time:** 5 minutes | **Cooking Time:** 45 minutes | **Serves:** 4

**Ingredients:**
- 1 teaspoon Chinese five spice powder
- 1 teaspoon white pepper
- 2 pounds pork belly
- 2 teaspoons garlic salt

**Directions:**
1. Preparing the Ingredients. Preheat the air fryer to 390°F.
2. Mix all of the seasonings in a bowl to create the dry rub.
3. Score the skin of the pork belly with a knife and season the entire pork with the spice rub.
4. Air Frying. Place in the air fryer and cook for 40 to 45 minutes until the skin is crispy.
5. Chop before serving.

Cal 785 | Fat 80.7g | Protein 14.2g

# Beef Rolls

**Preparation Time:** 10 minutes | **Cooking Time:** 14 minutes | **Serves:** 4

**Ingredients:**
- 2 pounds beef steak, opened and flattened with a meat tenderizer

- Salt and black pepper to the taste
- 3 ounces red bell pepper, roasted and chopped
- 6 slices provolone cheese
- 3 tablespoons pesto

**Directions:**

1. Arrange flattened beef steak on a cutting board, spread pesto all over, add cheese in a single layer, add bell peppers, salt and pepper to the taste.
2. Roll your steak, secure with toothpicks, season again with salt and pepper, place roll in your air fryer's basket and cook at 400°F for 14 minutes, rotating roll halfway.
3. Leave aside to cool down, cut into 2-inch smaller rolls, arrange on a platter and serve them as an appetizer.
4. Enjoy!

Cal 230 | Fat 1g |Fiber 3g | Carb 12g | Protein 10g

## Homemade Corned Beef with Onions

**Preparation Time:** 5 minutes | **Cooking Time:** 50 minutes | **Serves:** 4

**Ingredients:**

- Salt and pepper to taste
- 1 cup water
- 1-pound corned beef brisket, cut into chunks
- 1 tablespoon Dijon mustard
- 1 small onion, chopped

**Directions:**

1. Preheat the air fryer to 400°F.
2. Place all ingredients in a baking dish that will fit in the air fryer.
3. Cover with foil.
4. Cook for 35 minutes.
5. Remove foil, mix well, turnover beef, and continue cooking for another 15 minutes.

Cal 238 | Carb 3.1g | Protein 17.2g | Fat 17.1g | Fiber 0.6g

## Roast Beef

**Preparation Time:** 10 minutes | **Cooking Time:** 35 minutes | **Serves:** 4

**Ingredients:**

- 2 lb. beef roast top
- oil for spraying

- Rub
- salt and pepper to taste
- 2 teaspoon garlic powder
- 1 teaspoon summer savory

**Directions:**
1. Whisk all the rub ingredients in a small bowl.
2. Liberally rub this mixture over the roast.
3. Place in the Air Fryer Basket and layer it with cooking oil.
4. Set the seasoned roast in the Air Fryer Basket.
5. Take to the preheated air fryer at 370°F for 20 minutes.
6. Turn the roast and continue Air fryer for another 15 minutes.
7. Serve warm.

Cal 427 | Fat 14.2g | Carb 1.4g | Fiber 0.3g | Protein 69.1g

# Beef Tenderloin

**Preparation Time:** 5 minutes | **Cooking Time:** 30 minutes | **Serves:** 6

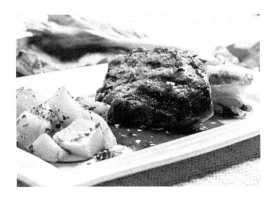

**Ingredients:**
- 1 (2-poundbeef tenderloin, trimmed of visible fat
- 2 tbsp. salted butter; melted.
- 2 tsp. minced roasted garlic
- 3 tbsp. ground 4-peppercorn blend

**Directions:**
1. In a small bowl, mix the butter and roasted garlic. Brush it over the beef tenderloin.
2. Place the ground peppercorns onto a plate and roll the tenderloin through them, creating a crust. Place tenderloin into your Kalorik Maxx Air Fryer basket

3. Adjust the temperature to 400 Degrees F and set the timer for 25 minutes. Flip the tenderloin halfway through cooking. Set aside for 10 minutes before slicing.

Cal 289 | Protein 37g |Fiber 9g | Fat 18g | Carb 5g

## Breaded Pork Chops

**Preparation Time:** 10 minutes | **Cooking Time:** 18 minutes | **Serves:** 4

**Ingredients:**
- 4 boneless, center-cut pork chops, 1-inch thick
- 1 teaspoon Cajun seasoning
- 1 1/2 cups garlic-flavored croutons
- 2 eggs
- cooking spray

**Directions:**
1. Grind croutons in a food processor until it forms crumbs.
2. Season the pork chops with Cajun seasoning liberally.
3. Beat eggs in a shallow tray then dip the pork chops in the egg.
4. Coat the dipped chops in the crouton crumbs.
5. Spray the chops with cooking oil.
6. Take to the preheated air fryer at 380°F for 18 minutes.
7. Serve.

Cal 301 |Fat 12.4g | Carb 12.2g |Fiber 0g | Protein 32.2g

## Air Fryer Meatloaf

**Preparation Time:** 10 minutes | **Cooking Time:** 25 minutes | **Serves:** 4

**Ingredients:**
- 1-pound lean beef
- 1 lightly beaten egg
- 3 tablespoons. bread crumbs
- 1 small, finely chopped onion
- 1 tablespoon. chopped fresh thyme
- 1 teaspoon salt
- 1 pinch ground black pepper to taste
- 2 thickly sliced mushrooms
- 1 tablespoon. olive oil

**Directions:**
1. Preheat an air fryer up to 390°F.

2. In a bowl, combine ground beef, egg, bread crumbs, ointment, thyme, salt, and pepper. Knead and mix well.
3. Move the mixture of beef into a baking pan and smooth the rim—press chestnuts into the top and coat with olive oil. Place the saucepan in the basket of the air fryer and slide into your Kalorik Maxx Air Fryer.
4. Set 25-minute air fryer timer and roast meatloaf until well browned.
5. Set aside the meatloaf for at least 10 minutes before slicing and serving into wedges.

Cal 296.8 | Protein 24.8g |Carb 5.9 g

# Basic Pork Chops

**Preparation Time:** 10 minutes | **Cooking Time:** 15 minutes | **Serves:** 4

**Ingredients:**
- 4 pork chops, bone-in
- 1 tablespoon olive oil
- 1 teaspoon kosher salt
- 1/2 teaspoon black pepper

**Directions:**
1. Liberally season the pork chops with olive oil, salt, and black pepper.
2. Spray the chops with cooking oil.
3. Take to the preheated air fryer at 380°F for 15 minutes.
4. Serve.

Cal 287 |Fat 23.4g | Carb 0.2g | Fiber 0.1g | Protein 18g

# Beef and Balsamic Marinade

**Preparation Time:** 5 minutes | **Cooking Time:** 40 minutes | **Serves:** 4

**Ingredients:**
- 4 medium beef steaks
- 3 garlic cloves; minced
- 1 cup balsamic vinegar
- 2 tbsp. olive oil
- Salt and black pepper to taste.

**Directions:**
1. Take a bowl and mix steaks with the rest of the ingredients and toss.
2. Transfer the steaks to your air fryer's basket and cook at 390°F for 35 minutes, flipping them halfway
3. Divide among plates and serve with a side salad.

Cal 273 | Fat 14g |Fiber 4g | Carb 6g | Protein 19g

## Honey Mustard
## Pork Tenderloin

**Preparation Time:** 15 minutes | **Cooking Time**: 25 minutes | **Serves:** 3

**Ingredients:**

- 1-pound pork tenderloin
- 1 tablespoon garlic, minced
- 2 tablespoons soy sauce
- 2 tablespoons honey
- 1 tablespoon Dijon mustard
- 1 tablespoon grain mustard
- 1 teaspoon Sriracha sauce

**Directions:**

1. In a large bowl, add all the ingredients except pork and mix well.
2. Add the pork tenderloin and coat with the mixture generously.
3. Refrigerate to marinate for 2-3 hours.
4. Remove the pork tenderloin from bowl, reserving the marinade.
5. Place the pork tenderloin onto the lightly greased cooking tray.
6. Arrange the drip pan in the bottom of Air Fryer Oven cooking chamber.
7. Take to the preheated air fryer at 380°F for 25 minutes.
8. After 12 minutes When the display shows "Turn Food" turn the pork and oat with the reserved marinade.
9. When cooking time is complete, remove the tray from Air Fryer and place the pork tenderloin onto a platter for about 10 minutes before slicing.
10. With a sharp knife, cut the pork tenderloin into desired sized slices and serve.

Cal 277 |Fat 5.7g | Carb 14.2g |Fiber 0.4g | Sugar 11.8g | Protein 40.7 g

## Beef and Radishes

**Preparation Time:** 5 minutes | **Cooking Time:** 15 minutes | **Serves:** 2

**Ingredients:**

- 1 lb. radishes, quartered
- 2 cups corned beef, cooked and shredded
- 2 spring onions; chopped
- 2 garlic cloves; minced
- A pinch of salt and black pepper

**Directions:**

1. In a pan that fits your air fryer, mix the beef with the rest of the ingredients, toss.
2. Put the pan in the fryer and cook at 390°F for 15 minutes
3. Divide everything into bowls and serve.

Cal 267 | Fat 13g |Fiber 2g | Carb 5g | Protein 15g

## Crispy Brats

**Preparation Time:** 5 minutes | **Cooking Time:** 15 minutes | **Serves:** 4

**Ingredients:**
- 4 (3-oz. beef bratwursts

**Directions:**
1. Place brats into your Kalorik Maxx Air Fryer basket.
2. Adjust the temperature to 375 Degrees F and set the timer for 15 minutes.

Cal 286 | Protein 18g |Fiber 0g | Fat 28g | Carb 0g

## Basil Pork Chops

**Preparation Time:** 5 minutes | **Cooking Time:** 30 minutes | **Serves:** 4

**Ingredients:**
- 4 pork chops
- 2 tsp. basil; dried
- ½ tsp. chili powder
- 2 tbsp. olive oil
- A pinch of salt and black pepper

**Directions:**
1. In a pan that fits your air fryer, mix all the ingredients, toss.
2. Introduce in the fryer and cook at 400°F for 25 minutes. Divide everything between plates and serve

Cal 274 | Fat 13g |Fiber 4g | Carb 6g | Protein 18g

## Seasoned Pork Chops

**Preparation Time:** 10 minutes | **Cooking Time**: 12 minutes | **Serves:** 4

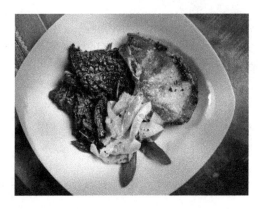

**Ingredients:**

- 4 (6-ounce) boneless pork chops
- 2 tablespoons pork rub
- 1 tablespoon olive oil

**Directions:**

1. Coat both sides of the pork chops with the oil and then, rub with the pork rub.
2. Place the pork chops onto the lightly greased cooking tray.
3. Arrange the drip pan in the bottom of Air Fryer Oven cooking chamber.
4. Take to the preheated air fryer at 400°F for 12 minutes in the center position.
5. After 6 minutes turn the pork chops.
6. When cooking time is complete, remove the tray from Air Fryer and serve hot.

Cal 285 | Fat 9.5g | Carb 1.5 g| Fiber 0 g| Sugar 0.8g | Protein 44.5 g

# Herbed Pork Chops

**Preparation Time:** 5 minutes | **Cooking Time:** 25 minutes | **Serves:** 4

**Ingredients:**

- 4 pork chops
- 2 tsp. basil; dried
- ½ tsp. chili powder
- 2 tbsp. olive oil
- A pinch of salt and black pepper

**Directions:**

1. In a pan that fits your air fryer, mix all the ingredients, toss.
2. Introduce in the fryer and cook at 400°F for 25 minutes. Divide everything between plates and serve

Cal 274 | Fat 13g |Fiber 4g | Carb 6g | Protein 18g

# Lamb Burgers

**Preparation Time:** 15 minutes | **Cooking Time**: 8 minutes | **Serves:** 6

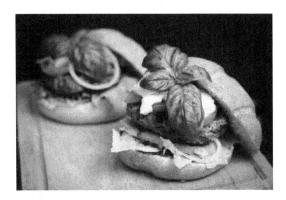

**Ingredients:**
- 2 pounds ground lamb
- 1 tablespoon onion powder
- Salt and ground black pepper, as required

**Directions:**
1. In a bowl, add all the ingredients and mix well.
2. Make 6 equal-sized patties from the mixture and arrange the patties onto a cooking tray.
3. Arrange the drip pan in the bottom of Air Fryer Oven cooking chamber.
4. Take to the preheated air fryer at 360°F for 8 minutes. Turn the burgers after 4 minutes.
5. When cooking time is complete, remove the tray from Air Fryer and serve hot.

Cal 285 | Fat 11.1g | Carb 0.9g | Fiber 0.1g | Sugar 0.4g | Protein 42.6 g

# Cajun Bacon Pork Loin Fillet

**Preparation Time:** 10 minutes | **Cooking Time**: 20 minutes | **Serves:** 6

**Ingredients:**
- 1½ pounds pork loin fillet or pork tenderloin
- 3 tablespoons olive oil
- 2 tablespoons Cajun Spice Mix
- Salt
- 6 slices bacon
- Olive oil spray

## Directions:

1. Preparing the Ingredients. Cut the pork in half so that it will fit in the air fryer basket.
2. Place both pieces of meat in a resealable plastic bag. Add the oil, Cajun seasoning, and salt to taste, if using. Seal the bag and massage to coat all of the meat with the oil and seasonings. Marinate in the refrigerator for at least 1 hour or up to 24 hours.
3. Air Frying. Remove the pork from the bag and wrap 3 bacon slices around each piece. Spray the air fryer basket with olive oil spray. Place the meat in the air fryer. Set the air fryer to 350°F for 15 minutes. Increase the temperature to 400°F for 5 minutes.
4. Use a meat thermometer to ensure the meat has reached an internal temperature of 145°F.
5. Let the meat rest for 10 minutes. Slice into 6 medallions and serve.

Cal 355Cal | Protein 34.83g | Fat 22.88 g| Carb 0.6 g

# Porchetta-Style Pork Chops

**Preparation Time:** 10 minutes | **Cooking Time**: 15 minutes | **Serves:** 2

## Ingredients:

- 1 tablespoon extra-virgin olive oil
- Grated zest of 1 lemon
- 2 cloves garlic, minced
- 2 teaspoons chopped fresh rosemary
- 1 teaspoon finely chopped fresh sage
- 1 teaspoon fennel seeds, lightly crushed
- ¼ to ½ teaspoon red pepper flakes
- 1 teaspoon kosher salt
- 1 teaspoon black pepper
- (8-ounce) center-cut bone-in pork chops, about 1 inch thick

## Directions:

1. Preparing the Ingredients. In a small bowl, combine the olive oil, zest, garlic, rosemary, sage, fennel seeds, red pepper, salt, and black pepper. Stir, crushing the herbs with the back of a spoon, until a paste forms. Spread the seasoning mix on both sides of the pork chops.
2. Air Frying. Place the chops in the air fryer basket. Set the air fryer to 375°F for 15 minutes. Use a meat thermometer to ensure the chops have reached an internal temperature of 145°F.

Cal 200Cal | Protein 23.45g | Fat 9.7g| Carb 4.46 g

## Apricot Glazed Pork Tenderloins

**Preparation Time:** 5 minutes | **Cooking Time**: 30 minutes | **Serves:** 3
**Ingredients:**
- 1 teaspoon salt
- 1/2 teaspoon pepper
- 1-lb pork tenderloin
- 2 tablespoons minced fresh rosemary or 1 tablespoon dried rosemary, crushed
- 2 tablespoons olive oil, divided
- 1 garlic cloves, minced
- Apricot Glaze Ingredients
- 1 cup apricot preserves
- 3 garlic cloves, minced
- 4 tablespoons lemon juice

**Directions:**
1. Preparing the Ingredients. Mix well pepper, salt, garlic, oil, and rosemary. Brush all over pork. If needed cut pork crosswise in half to fit in air fryer. Lightly grease baking pan of air fryer with cooking spray. Add pork.
2. Air Frying. For 3 minutes per side, brown pork in a preheated 390°F air fryer. Meanwhile, mix well all glaze Ingredients in a small bowl. Baste pork every 5 minutes. Cook for 20 minutes at 330°F. Serve and enjoy.

Cal 454Cal | Protein 43.76g | Fat 16.71 g| Carb 33.68 g

## Sweet & Spicy
## Country-Style Ribs

**Preparation Time:** 10 minutes | **Cooking Time**: 25 minutes | **Serves:** 4
**Ingredients:**
- 2 tablespoons brown sugar
- 2 tablespoons smoked paprika
- 1 teaspoon garlic powder
- 1 teaspoon onion powder
- 1 teaspoon dry mustard
- 1 teaspoon ground cumin
- 1 teaspoon kosher salt
- 1 teaspoon black pepper

- ¼ to ½ teaspoon cayenne pepper
- 1½ pounds boneless country-style pork ribs
- 1 cup barbecue sauce

**Directions:**
1. Preparing the Ingredients. In a small bowl, stir together the brown sugar, paprika, garlic powder, onion powder, dry mustard, cumin, salt, black pepper, and cayenne. Mix until well combined.
2. Pat the ribs dry with a paper towel. Generously sprinkle the rub evenly over both sides of the ribs and rub in with your fingers.
3. Air Frying. Place the ribs in the air fryer basket. Set the air fryer to 350°F for 15 minutes. Turn the ribs and brush with ½ cup of the barbecue sauce. Cook for an additional 10 minutes. Use a meat thermometer to ensure the pork has reached an internal temperature of 145°F. Serve with remaining barbecue sauce.

Cal 416Cal | Protein 38.39g | Fat 12.19 g| Carb 36.79 g

# Flavorful steak

**Preparation Time:** 10 minutes | **Cooking Time**: 18 minutes | **Serves:** 2

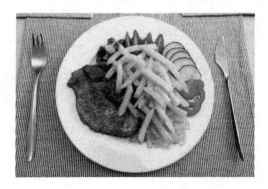

**Ingredients:**
- 2 steaks, rinsed and pat dry
- ½ tsp garlic powder
- 1 tsp olive oil
- Pepper
- Salt

**Directions:**
1. Brush steaks with olive oil and season with garlic powder, pepper, and salt.
2. Preheat the Air Fryer oven to 400°F.

3. Place steaks on air fryer oven pan and air fry for 10-18 minutes. Turn halfway through.
4. Serve and enjoy.

Cal 361 | Fat 10.9g | Carb 0.5g | Sugar 0.2g | Protein 61.6 g

# Pork Tenders with Bell Peppers

**Preparation Time:** 5 minutes | **Cooking Time**: 15 minutes | **Serves:** 4

**Ingredients:**
- 11 Oz Pork Tenderloin
- 1 Bell Pepper, in thin strips
- 1 Red Onion, sliced
- 2 Tsps. Provencal Herbs
- Black Pepper to taste
- 1 tbsp. Olive Oil
- 1/2 tbsp. Mustard

**Directions:**
1. Preparing the Ingredients. Preheat the air fryer to 390°F.
2. In the oven dish, mix the bell pepper strips with the onion, herbs, and some salt and pepper to taste.
3. Add half a tablespoon of olive oil to the mixture
4. Cut the pork tenderloin into four pieces and rub with salt, pepper and mustard.
5. Thinly coat the pieces with remaining olive oil and place them upright in the oven dish on top of the pepper mixture
6. Air Frying. Place the bowl into your Kalorik Maxx Air Fryer. Set the timer to 15 minutes and cook the meat and the vegetables
7. Turn the meat and mix the peppers halfway through
8. Serve with a fresh salad

Cal 220Cal | Protein 23.79g | Fat 12.36 g| Carb 2.45 g

# Wonton Meatballs

**Preparation Time:** 15 minutes | **Cooking Time**: 10 minutes | **Serves:** 4

**Ingredients:**
- 1-pound ground pork
- 2 large eggs
- ¼ cup chopped green onions (white and green parts)
- ¼ cup chopped fresh cilantro or parsley
- 1 tablespoon minced fresh ginger

- 3 cloves garlic, minced
- 2 teaspoons soy sauce
- 1 teaspoon oyster sauce
- ½ teaspoon kosher salt
- 1 teaspoon black pepper

**Directions:**

1. Preparing the Ingredients. In the bowl of a stand mixer fitted with the paddle attachment, combine the pork, eggs, green onions, cilantro, ginger, garlic, soy sauce, oyster sauce, salt, and pepper. Mix on low speed until all of the ingredients are incorporated, 2 to 3 minutes.
2. Form the mixture into 12 meatballs and arrange in a single layer in the air fryer basket.
3. Air Frying. Set the air fryer to 350°F for 10 minutes. Use a meat thermometer to ensure the meatballs have reached an internal temperature of 145°F.
4. Transfer the meatballs to a bowl and serve.

Cal 402Cal | Protein 32.69g | Fat 27.91 g| Carb 3.1 g

## Chopped Bondiola

**Preparation Time:** 5 minutes | **Cooking Time:** 10 minutes | **Serves:** 4

**Ingredients:**

- 1kg Bondiola in pieces
- Bread crumbs
- two eggs
- Seasoning to taste

**Directions:**

1. Cut the bondiola into small pieces, seasonings to taste.
2. Beat the eggs.
3. Passe the bondiola seasoned by beaten egg and then by breadcrumbs.
4. Then we place in the air fryer for 20 minutes, in half time we turn and snacks of bondiola ready.

Cal 140 | Fat 4g | Carb 7g | Protein 11g

## Barbecue Flavored Pork Ribs

**Preparation Time:** 5 minutes | **Cooking Time:**15 minutes | **Serves:** 6

**Ingredients:**

- ¼ cup honey, divided
- ¾ cup BBQ sauce

- 2 tablespoons tomato ketchup
- 1 tablespoon Worcestershire sauce
- 1 tablespoon soy sauce
- ½ teaspoon garlic powder
- Freshly ground white pepper, to taste
- 1¾ pound pork ribs

**Directions:**

1. Preparing the ingredients. In a large bowl, mix together 3 tablespoons of honey and remaining ingredients except pork ribs. Refrigerate to marinate for about 20 minutes. Preheat the air fryer to 355°F. Place the ribs in the Air fryer basket.
2. Air Frying. Cook for about 13 minutes. Remove the ribs from the Air fryer and coat with remaining honey. Serve hot.

Cal 265Cal | Protein 29.47g | Fat 9.04 g| Carb 15.87 g

# Marinated Pork Tenderloin

**Preparation Time:** 1 hour & 10 minutes | **Cooking Time**: 30 minutes | **Serves:** 4

**Ingredients:**

- ¼ cup olive oil
- ¼ cup soy sauce
- ¼ cup freshly squeezed lemon juice
- 1 garlic clove, minced
- 1 tablespoon Dijon mustard
- 1 teaspoon salt
- ½ teaspoon freshly ground black pepper
- 2 pounds pork tenderloin

**Directions:**

1. Preparing the Ingredients. In a large mixing bowl, make the marinade. Mix together the olive oil, soy sauce, lemon juice, minced garlic, Dijon mustard, salt, and pepper. Reserve ¼ cup of the marinade.
2. Place the tenderloin in a large bowl and pour the remaining marinade over the meat. Cover and marinate in the refrigerator for about 1 hour. Place the marinated pork tenderloin into your Kalorik Maxx Air Fryer basket.
3. Set the temperature to 400°F. Set the timer and roast for 10 minutes. Using tongs, flip the pork and baste it with half of the reserved marinade. Reset the timer and roast for 10 minutes more.
4. Using tongs, flip the pork, then baste with the remaining marinade.
5. Reset the timer and roast for another 10 minutes, for a total cooking time of 30 minutes.

Cal 345Cal | Protein 41.56g | Fat 17.35 g| Carb 3.66 g

# Poultry recipes

## BBQ Chicken Breasts

**Preparation Time:** 5 minutes | **Cooking Time:** 15 minutes | **Serves:** 4

**Ingredients:**
- Boneless, skinless chicken breast – 4, about 6 oz. each
- BBQ seasoning – 2 tbsps.
- Cooking spray

**Directions:**
1. Rub the chicken with BBQ seasoning and marinate in the refrigerator for 45 minutes. Preheat the air fryer at 400°F. Grease the basket with oil and place the chicken.
2. Then spray oil on top. Cook for 13 to 14 minutes. Flipping at the halfway mark. Serve.

Cal 131 | Carb 2g | Fat 3g | Protein 24g

## Buffalo Chicken Tenders

**Preparation Time:** 5 minutes | **Cooking Time:** 20 minutes | **Serves:** 4

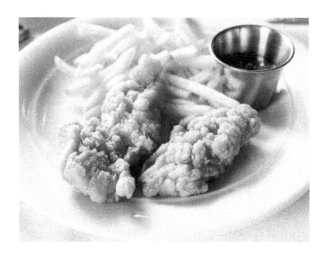

**Ingredients:**
- Boneless, skinless chicken tenders – 1 pound
- Hot sauce – ¼ cup
- Pork rinds – 1 ½ ounces, finely ground
- Chili powder – 1 tsp.
- Garlic powder – 1 tsp.

**Directions:**
1. Put the chicken breasts in a bowl and pour hot sauce over them. Toss to coat. Mix ground pork rinds, chili powder and garlic powder in another bowl.
2. Place each tender in the ground pork rinds, and coat well. With wet hands, press down the pork rinds into the chicken. Place the tender in a single layer into your Kalorik Maxx Air Fryer basket. Cook at 375°F for 20 minutes. Flip once. Serve.

Cal 160 | Carb 0.6g | Fat 4.4g | Protein 27.3g

## Rotisserie Chicken

**Preparation Time:** 5 minutes | **Cooking Time:** 1 hour | **Serves:** 4

**Ingredients:**
- Whole chicken – 1, cleaned and patted dry
- Olive oil – 2 tbsps.
- Seasoned salt – 1 tbsp.

**Directions:**
1. Remove the giblet packet from the cavity. Rub the chicken with oil and salt. Place in the air fryer basket, breast-side down. Cook at 350°F for 30 minutes.
2. Then flip and cook another 30 minutes. Chicken is done when it reaches 165°F.

Cal 534 | Carb 0g | Fat 36g | Protein 35g

# Honey-Mustard Chicken Breasts

**Preparation Time:** 5 minutes | **Cooking Time:** 25 minutes | **Serves:** 6

**Ingredients:**
- Boneless, skinless chicken breasts – 6 (6-oz, each)
- Fresh rosemary – 2 tbsps. minced
- Honey – 3 tbsps.
- Dijon mustard – 1 tbsp.
- Salt and pepper to taste

**Directions:**
1. Combine the mustard, honey, pepper, rosemary and salt in a bowl. Rub the chicken with this mixture.
2. Grease the air fryer basket with oil. Air fry the chicken at 350°F for 20 to 24 minutes or until the chicken reaches 165°F. Serve.

Cal 236 | Carb 9.8g | Fat 5g | Protein 38g

# Chicken Parmesan Wings

**Preparation Time:** 5 minutes | **Cooking Time:** 15 minutes | **Serves:** 4

**Ingredients:**
- Chicken wings – 2 lbs. cut into drumettes, pat dried
- Parmesan – ½ cup, plus 6 tbsps. grated
- Herbs de Provence – 1 tsp.
- Paprika – 1 tsp.
- Salt to taste

**Directions:**
1. Combine the parmesan, herbs, paprika, and salt in a bowl and rub the chicken with this mixture. Preheat the air fryer at 350°F.
2. Grease the basket with cooking spray. Cook for 15 minutes. Flip once at the halfway mark. Garnish with parmesan and serve.

Cal 490 | Carb 1g | Fat 22g | Protein 72g

# Air Fryer Chicken

**Preparation Time:** 5 minutes | **Cooking Time:** 30 minutes | **Serves:** 4

**Ingredients:**
- Chicken wings – 2 lbs.
- Salt and pepper to taste
- Cooking spray

**Directions:**

1. Flavor the chicken wings with salt and pepper. Grease the air fryer basket with cooking spray. Add chicken wings and cook at 400°F for 35 minutes.
2. Flip 3 times during cooking for even cooking. Serve.

Cal 277 | Carb 1g | Fat 8g | Protein 50g

## Whole Chicken

**Preparation Time:** 5 minutes | **Cooking Time:** 40 minutes | **Serves:** 6

**Ingredients:**

- Whole chicken – 1 (2 ½ pounds) washed and pat dried
- Dry rub – 2 tbsps.
- Salt – 1 tsp.
- Cooking spray

**Directions:**

1. Preheat the air fryer at 350°F. Rub the dry rub on the chicken. Then rub with salt. Cook it at 350°F for 45 minutes. After 30 minutes, flip the chicken and finish cooking.
2. Chicken is done when it reaches 165°F.

Cal 412 | Carb 1g | Fat 28g | Protein 35g

## Honey Duck Breasts

**Preparation Time:** 5 minutes | **Cooking Time:** 25 minutes | **Serves:** 2

**Ingredients:**

- Smoked duck breast – 1, halved
- Honey – 1 tsp.
- Tomato paste – 1 tsp.
- Mustard – 1 tbsp.
- Apple vinegar – ½ tsp.

**Directions:**

1. Mix tomato paste, honey, mustard, and vinegar in a bowl. Whisk well. Add duck breast pieces and coat well. Cook in the air fryer at 370°F for 15 minutes.
2. Remove the duck breast from the air fryer and add to the honey mixture. Coat again. Cook again at 370°F for 6 minutes. Serve.

Cal 274 | Carb 22g | Fat 11g | Protein 13g

# Creamy Coconut Chicken

**Preparation Time:** 5 minutes | **Cooking Time:** 20 minutes | **Serves:** 4

**Ingredients:**

- Big chicken legs – 4
- Turmeric powder – 5 tsps.
- Ginger – 2 tbsps. grated
- Salt and black pepper to taste
- Coconut cream – 4 tbsps.

**Directions:**

1. In a bowl, mix salt, pepper, ginger, turmeric, and cream. Whisk. Add chicken pieces, coat and marinate for 2 hours.
2. Transfer chicken to the preheated air fryer and cook at 370°F for 25 minutes. Serve.

Cal 300 | Carb 22g | Fat 4g | Protein 20g

# Teriyaki Wings

**Preparation Time:** 5 minutes | **Cooking Time:** 20 minutes | **Serves:** 4

**Ingredients:**

- Chicken wings – 2 pounds
- Teriyaki sauce – ½ cup
- Minced garlic – 2 tsp.
- Ground ginger - ¼ tsp.
- Baking powder – 2 tsp.

**Directions:**

1. Except for the baking powder, place all ingredients in a bowl and marinate for 1 hour in the refrigerator. Place wings into your Kalorik Maxx Air Fryer basket and sprinkle with baking powder.
2. Gently rub into wings. Cook at 400°F for 25 minutes. Shake the basket two- or three-times during cooking. Serve.

Cal 446 | Carb 3.1g | Fat 29.8g | Protein 41.8g

# Lemony Drumsticks

**Preparation Time:** 5 minutes | **Cooking Time:** 20 minutes | **Serves:** 2

**Ingredients:**

- Baking powder – 2 tsps.
- Garlic powder – ½ tsp.
- Chicken drumsticks – 8
- Salted butter – 4 tbsps. melted
- Lemon pepper seasoning – 1 tbsp.

**Directions:**
1. Sprinkle garlic powder and baking powder over drumsticks and rub into chicken skin. Place drumsticks into your Kalorik Maxx Air Fryer basket. Cook at 375°F for 25 minutes. Flip the drumsticks once halfway through the Cooking Time.
2. Remove when cooked. Mix seasoning and butter in a bowl. Add drumsticks to the bowl and toss to coat. Serve.

Cal 532 | Carb 1.2g | Fat 32.3g | Protein 48.3g

# Parmesan Chicken Tenders

**Preparation Time:** 5 minutes | **Cooking Time:** 10 minutes | **Serves:** 4

**Ingredients:**
- 1 pound chicken tenderloins
- 3 large egg whites
- ½ cup Italian-style bread crumbs
- ¼ cup grated Parmesan cheese

**Directions:**
1. Preparing the Ingredients. Spray the air fryer basket with olive oil. Trim off any white fat from the chicken tenders. In a bowl, whisk the egg whites until frothy. In a separate small mixing bowl, combine the bread crumbs and Parmesan cheese. Mix well.
2. Dip the chicken tenders into the egg mixture, then into the Parmesan and bread crumbs. Shake off any excess breading. Place the chicken tenders in the greased air fryer basket in a single layer. Generously spray the chicken with olive oil to avoid powdery, uncooked breading.
3. Set the temperature of your Air Fryer to 370°F. Set the timer and bake for 4 minutes. Using tongs, flip the chicken tenders and bake for 4 minutes more. Check that the chicken has reached an internal temperature of 165°F. Add Cooking Time if needed. Once the chicken is fully cooked, plate, serve, and enjoy.

Cal 210 | Fat 4g |Carb 10g | Fiber 1g | Sugar 1g | Protein 33g

# Easy Lemon Chicken Thighs

**Preparation Time:** 5 minutes | **Cooking Time:** 10 minutes | **Serves:** 4

**Ingredients:**

- Salt and black pepper to taste
- 2 tablespoons olive oil
- 2 tablespoons Italian seasoning
- 2 tablespoons freshly squeezed lemon juice
- 1 lemon, sliced

**Directions:**

1. Place the chicken thighs in a medium mixing bowl and season them with the salt and pepper. Add the olive oil, Italian seasoning, and lemon juice and toss until the chicken thighs are thoroughly coated with oil. Add the sliced lemons. Place the chicken thighs into your Kalorik Maxx Air Fryer basket in a single layer.
2. Set the temperature of your Air Fryer to 350°F. Set the timer and cook for 10 minutes. Using tongs, flip the chicken. Reset the timer and cook for 10 minutes more. Check that the chicken has reached an internal temperature of 165°F. Add Cooking Time if needed.
3. Once the chicken is fully cooked, plate, serve, and enjoy.

Cal 325 | Carb 1g | Fat 26g | Protein 20g

# Air Fryer Grilled Chicken Breasts

**Preparation Time:** 5 minutes | **Cooking Time:** 14 minutes | **Serves:** 4

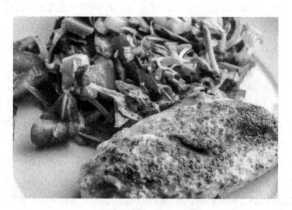

**Ingredients:**

- ½ teaspoon garlic powder
- salt and black pepper to taste
- 1 teaspoon dried parsley
- 2 tablespoons olive oil, divided

- 3 boneless, skinless chicken breasts

**Directions:**
1. Preparing the Ingredients. In a small bowl, combine together the garlic powder, salt, pepper, and parsley. Using 1 tablespoon of olive oil and half of the seasoning mix, rub each chicken breast with oil and seasonings. Place the chicken breast in the air fryer basket.
2. Set the temperature of your Air Fryer to 370°F. Set the timer and grill for 7 minutes.
3. Using tongs, flip the chicken and brush the remaining olive oil and spices onto the chicken. Reset the timer and grill for 7 minutes more. Check that the chicken has reached an internal temperature of 165°F. Add Cooking Time if needed.
4. When the chicken is cooked, transfer it to a platter and serve.

Cal 182 | Carb 0g | Fat 9g | Protein 26g

## Crispy Air Fryer Butter Chicken

**Preparation Time:** 5 minutes | **Cooking Time:** 15 minutes | **Serves:** 4

**Ingredients:**
- 2 (8-ounce) boneless, skinless chicken breasts
- 1 sleeve Ritz crackers
- 4 tablespoons (½ stick) cold unsalted butter, cut into 1-tablespoon slices

**Directions:**
1. Preparing the Ingredients. Spray the air fryer basket with olive oil, or spray an air fryer–size baking sheet with olive oil or cooking spray.
2. Dip the chicken breasts in water. Put the crackers in a resealable plastic bag. Using a mallet or your hands, crush the crackers. Place the chicken breasts inside the bag one at a time and coat them with the cracker crumbs.
3. Place the chicken in the greased air fryer basket, or on the greased baking sheet set into your Kalorik Maxx Air Fryer basket. Put 1 to 2 dabs of butter onto each piece of chicken.
4. Set the temperature of your Air Fryer to 370°F. Set the timer and bake for 7 minutes.
5. Using tongs, flip the chicken. Spray the chicken generously with olive oil to avoid uncooked breading. Reset the timer and bake for 7 minutes more.
6. Check that the chicken has reached an internal temperature of 165°F. Add Cooking Time if needed. Using tongs, remove the chicken from the air fryer and serve.

Cal 750 | Fat 40g | Carb 38g | Protein 57g

# Light and Airy Breaded Chicken Breasts

**Preparation Time:** 5 minutes | **Cooking Time:** 15 minutes | **Serves:** 2

**Ingredients:**
- 2 large eggs
- 1 cup bread crumbs or panko bread crumbs
- 1 teaspoon Italian seasoning
- 4 to 5 tablespoons vegetable oil
- 2 boneless, skinless, chicken breasts

**Directions:**
1. Preparing the Ingredients. Preheat the air fryer to 370°F. Spray the air fryer basket with olive oil or cooking spray. In a small bowl, whisk the eggs until frothy. In a separate small mixing bowl, mix together the bread crumbs, Italian seasoning, and oil. Dip the chicken in the egg mixture, then in the bread crumb mixture. Place the chicken directly into the greased air fryer basket, or on the greased baking sheet set into the basket.
2. Air Frying. Spray the chicken generously and thoroughly with olive oil to avoid powdery, uncooked breading. Set the timer and fry for 7 minutes. Using tongs, flip the chicken and generously spray it with olive oil. Reset the timer and fry for 7 minutes more. Check that the chicken has reached an internal temperature of 165°F. Add Cooking Time if needed. Once the chicken is fully cooked, use tongs to remove it from the air fryer and serve.

Cal 833 | Fat 46g | Carb 40g | Protein 65g

# Chicken Meatballs

**Preparation Time:** 5 minutes | **Cooking Time:** 15 minutes | **Serves:** 2

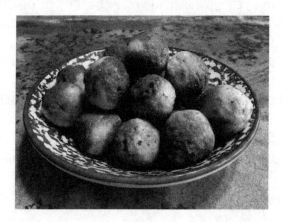

**Ingredients:**
- ½ lb chicken breast
- 1 tbsp of garlic
- 1 tbsp of onion
- ½ chicken broth
- 1 tbsp of oatmeal, whole wheat flour or of your choice

**Directions:**
1. Place all of the ingredients in a food processor and beat well until well mixed and ground.
2. If you don't have a food processor, ask the butcher to grind it and then add the other ingredients, mixing well.
3. Make balls and place them in the Air Fryer basket.
4. Program the Air Fryer for 15 minutes at 400ºF.
5. Half the time shake the basket so that the meatballs loosen and fry evenly.

Cal 45 | Carb 1.94g | Fat 1.57g | Protein 5.43g

## Chicken Fillets, Brie & Ham

**Preparation Time:** 5 minutes | **Cooking Time:** 15 minutes | **Serves:** 4

**Ingredients:**
- 2 Large Chicken Fillets
- Freshly Ground Black Pepper
- 4 Small Slices of Brie (Or your cheese of choice)
- 1 Tbsp Freshly Chopped Chives
- 4 Slices Cured Ham

**Directions:**
1. Preparing the Ingredients. Slice the fillets into four and make incisions as you would for a hamburger bun. Leave a little "hinge" uncut at the back. Season the inside and pop some brie and chives in there. Close them, and wrap them each in a slice of ham. Brush with oil and pop them into the basket.
2. Heat your fryer to 350°F. Roast the little parcels until they look tasty (15 min)

Cal 850 | Carb 43g | Fat 50g | Protein 76 g

## Air Fryer Cornish Hen

**Preparation Time:** 5 minutes | **Cooking Time:** 30 minutes | **Serves:** 2

**Ingredients:**
- 2 tablespoons Montreal chicken seasoning
- 1 (1½- to 2-pound) Cornish hen

**Directions:**

1. Preheat the air fryer to 390°F. Rub the seasoning over the chicken, coating it thoroughly.
2. Put the chicken in the basket. Set the timer and roast for 15 minutes.
3. Flip the chicken and cook for another 15 minutes. Check that the chicken has reached an internal temperature of 165°F. Add Cooking Time if needed.

Cal 520 | Fat 36g | Carb 0g | Protein 45g

# Air Fried Turkey Wings

**Preparation Time:** 5 minutes | **Cooking Time:** 26 minutes | **Serves:** 4

**Ingredients:**

- 2 pounds turkey wings
- 3 tablespoons olive oil or sesame oil
- 3 to 4 tablespoons chicken rub

**Directions:**

1. Put the turkey wings in a large mixing bowl. Pour the olive oil into the bowl and add the rub. Using your hands, rub the oil mixture over the turkey wings. Place the turkey wings in the air fryer basket.
2. Fix the temperature of your Air Fryer to 380°F. Set the timer and roast for 13 minutes.
3. Using tongs, flip the wings. Reset the timer and roast for 13 minutes more. Remove the turkey wings from the air fryer, plate, and serve.

Cal 521 | Fat 34g |Carb 4g | Protein 52g

# Chicken-Fried Steak Supreme

**Preparation Time:** 10 minutes | **Cooking Time:** 30 minutes | **Serves:** 8

**Ingredients:**

- ½ pound beef-bottom round, sliced into strips
- 1 cup of breadcrumbs
- 2 medium-sized eggs
- Pinch of salt and pepper
- ½ tablespoon of ground thyme

**Directions:**

1. Preparing the Ingredients. Cover the basket of the Air fryer with a layer of tin foil, leaving the edges open to allow air to flow through the basket. Preheat the air fryer to 350°F. In a bowl, whisk the eggs until fluffy and until the yolks and whites are fully combined, and set aside. In a separate bowl, mix the breadcrumbs,

thyme, salt and pepper, and set aside. One by one, dip each piece of raw steak into the bowl with dry ingredients, coating all sides; then submerge into the bowl with wet ingredients, then dip again into the dry ingredients. This double coating will ensure an extra crisp air fry. Lay the coated steak pieces on the foil covering the air-fryer basket, in a single flat layer.

2. Set the air fryer timer for 15 minutes. After 15 minutes, the air fryer will turn off and the steak should be mid-way cooked and the breaded coating starting to brown. Using tongs, turn each piece of steak over to ensure a full all-over fry. Reset the air fryer to 320 ° for 15 minutes. After 15 minutes, when the air fryer shuts off, remove the fried steak strips using tongs and set on a serving plate. Eat once cool enough to handle and enjoy.

Cal 421 | Fat 26g | Carb 8g | Protein 46g

## Caesar Marinated Grilled Chicken

**Preparation Time:** 10 minutes | **Cooking Time:** 25 minutes | **Serves:** 4

**Ingredients:**
- ¼ cup crouton
- 1 teaspoon lemon zest. Form into ovals, skewer and grill.
- 1/2 cup Parmesan
- 1/4 cup breadcrumbs
- 1-pound ground chicken
- 2 tablespoons Caesar dressing and more for drizzling
- 2-4 romaine leaves

**Directions:**
1. In a shallow dish, mix well chicken, 2 tablespoons Caesar dressing, parmesan, and breadcrumbs. Mix well with hands. Form into 1-inch oval patties. Thread chicken pieces in skewers. Place on skewer rack in air fryer.
2. For 12 minutes, cook on 360°F. Halfway through Cooking Time, turnover skewers. If needed, cook in batches. Serve on a bed of lettuce and sprinkle with croutons and extra dressing.

Cal 342 | Fat 12g | Carb 8g | Protein 36g

## Cheesy Chicken Tenders

**Preparation Time:** 10 minutes | **Cooking Time:** 30 minutes | **Serves:** 4

**Ingredients:**
- 1 large white meat chicken breast
- 1 cup of breadcrumbs

- 2 medium-sized eggs
- Pinch of salt and pepper
- 1 tablespoon of grated or powdered parmesan cheese

**Directions:**
1. Cover the basket of the Air fryer with a layer of tin foil, leaving the edges open to allow air to flow through the basket.
2. Preheat the air fryer to 350°F.
3. In a bowl, whisk the eggs until fluffy and until the yolks and whites are fully combined, and set aside. In a separate bowl, mixt he breadcrumbs, parmesan, salt and pepper, and set aside. One by one, dip each piece of raw chicken into the bowl with dry ingredients, coating all sides; then submerge into the bowl with wet ingredients, then dip again into the dry ingredients. Put the coated chicken pieces on the foil covering the Air fryer basket, in a single flat layer.
4. Set the air fryer timer for 15 minutes.
5. After 15 minutes, the air fryer will turn off and the chicken should be mid-way cooked and the breaded coating starting to brown. Flip each piece of chicken over to ensure a full all over fry.
6. Reset the air fryer to 320°F for another 15 minutes. After 15 minutes, when the air fryer shuts off, remove the fried chicken strips using tongs and set on a serving plate. Eat once cool enough to handle, and enjoy.

Cal 278 | Fat 15g | Protein 29g | Sugar 7g

---

# Mustard Chicken Tenders

**Preparation Time:** 5 minutes | **Cooking Time:** 20 minutes | **Serves:** 4

**Ingredients:**
- ½ C. coconut flour
- 1 tbsp. spicy brown mustard
- 2 beaten eggs
- 1 pound of chicken tenders

**Directions:**
1. Season tenders with pepper and salt.
2. Place a thin layer of mustard onto tenders and then dredge in flour and dip in egg.
3. Add to your Kalorik Maxx Air Fryer, set temperature to 390°F, and set time to 20 minutes.

Cal 346 | Fat 10g | Carb 12g | Protein 31g

# Barbecue with Chorizo and Chicken

**Preparation Time:** 5 minutes | **Cooking Time:** 35 minutes | **Serves:** 4

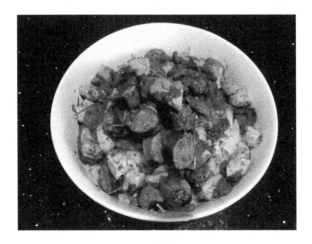

**Ingredients:**

- 4 chicken thighs
- 2 Tuscan sausages
- small onions

**Directions:**

1. Preheat the fryer to 400°F for 5 minutes. Season the meat the same way you would if you were going to use the barbecue.
2. Put in the fryer, lower the temperature to 320°C and set for 30 minutes.
3. After 20 minutes, check if any of the meat has reached the point of your preference. If so, take whichever is ready and return to the fryer with the others for another 10 minutes, now at 400°F. If not, return them to Air Fryer for the last 10 minutes at 400°F.

Cal 135 | Carb 0g | Fat 5g | Protein 6g

# Minty Chicken-Fried Pork Chops

**Preparation Time:** 10 minutes | **Cooking Time:** 30 minutes | **Serves:** 4

**Ingredients:**

- 4medium-sized pork chops
- 1 cup of breadcrumbs
- 2 medium-sized eggs
- Pinch of salt and pepper

- ½ tablespoon of mint, either dried and ground; or fresh, rinsed, and finely chopped

**Directions:**

1. Preparing the Ingredients. Cover the basket of the Air fryer with a layer of tin foil, leaving the edges open to allow air to flow through the basket.
2. Preheat the air fryer to 350°F. In a mixing bowl, whisk the eggs until fluffy and until the yolks and whites are fully combined, and set aside. In a separate bowl, mix the breadcrumbs, mint, salt and pepper, and set aside.
3. One by one, dip each raw pork chop into the bowl with dry ingredients, coating all sides; then submerge into the bowl with wet ingredients, then dip again into the dry ingredients. Lay the coated pork chops on the foil covering the Air fryer basket, in a single flat layer.
4. Set the air fryer timer for 15 minutes.
5. After 15 minutes, the Air fryer will turn off and the pork should be mid-way cooked and the breaded coating starting to brown. Using tongs, turn each piece of steak over to ensure a full all-over fry.
6. Reset the air fryer to 320°F for 15 minutes. After 15 minutes remove the fried pork chops using tongs and set on a serving plate.

Cal 262 | Fat 17g | Carb 7g | Protein 32g

## Breaded Nugget in Doritos

**Preparation Time:** 10 minutes | **Cooking Time:** 15 minutes | **Serves:** 4

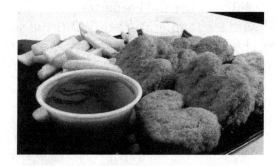

**Ingredients:**

- ½ lb. boneless, skinless chicken breast
- ¼ lb. Doritos snack
- 1 cup of wheat flour
- 1 egg
- Salt, garlic and black pepper to taste.

**Directions:**

1. Cut the chicken breast in the width direction, 1 to 1.5 cm thick, so that it is already shaped like pips.
2. Season with salt, garlic, black pepper to taste and some other seasonings if desired.
3. You can also season with those seasonings or powdered onion soup.
4. Put the Doritos snack in a food processor or blender and beat until everything is crumbled, but don't beat too much, you don't want flour.
5. Now bread, passing the pieces of chicken breast first in the wheat flour, then in the beaten eggs and finally in the Doritos, without leaving the excess flour, eggs or Doritos.
6. Place the seeds in the Air Fryer basket and program for 15 minutes at 400ºF, and half the time they brown evenly.

Cal 42 | Carb 1.65g | Fat 1.44g | Protein 5.29g | Sugar 0.1g

# Bacon Lovers' Stuffed Chicken

**Preparation Time:** 10 minutes | **Cooking Time:** 20 minutes | **Serves:** 4

**Ingredients:**
- 4 (5-ounce) boneless, skinless chicken breasts, sliced into ¼ inch thick
- 2 packages Boursin cheese
- 8 slices thin-cut bacon or beef bacon
- Sprig of fresh cilantro, for garnish

**Directions:**
1. Preparing the Ingredients. Spray the air fryer basket with avocado oil.
2. Preheat the air fryer to 400°F. Put one of the chicken breasts on a cutting board. With a sharp knife held parallel to the cutting board, make a 1-inch-wide incision at the top of the breast.
3. Carefully cut into the breast to form a large pocket, leaving a ½-inch border along the sides and bottom. Repeat with the other 3 chicken breasts. Snip the corner of a large resealable plastic bag to form a ¾-inch hole. Place the Boursin cheese in the bag and pipe the cheese into the pockets in the chicken breasts, dividing the cheese evenly among them. Wrap 2 slices of bacon around each chicken breast and secure the ends with toothpicks.
4. Air Frying. Place the bacon-wrapped chicken in the air fryer basket and cook until the bacon is crisp and the chicken's internal temperature reaches 165°F, about 18 to 20 minutes, flipping after 10 minutes.
5. Garnish with a sprig of cilantro before serving, if desired.

Cal 446 | Fat 17g | Carb 13g | Protein 36g

# Air Fryer Turkey Breast

**Preparation Time:** 5 minutes | **Cooking Time:** 60 minutes | **Serves:** 6

**Ingredients:**
- Pepper and salt
- 1 oven-ready turkey breast
- Turkey seasonings of choice

**Directions:**
1. Preheat the air fryer to 350°F.
2. Season turkey with pepper, salt, and other desired seasonings.
3. Place turkey in air fryer basket.
4. Set temperature to 350°F, and set time to 60 minutes. Cook 60 minutes. The meat should be at 165°F when done. Allow to rest 10-15 minutes before slicing. Enjoy.

Cal 212 | Fat 12g | Protein 24g | Sugar 0g

# Breaded Chicken without Flour

**Preparation Time:** 10 minutes | **Cooking Time:** 15 minutes | **Serves:** 6

**Ingredients:**
- 1 1/6 oz. of grated parmesan cheese
- 1 unit of egg
- 1 lb of chicken (breast)
- Salt and black pepper to taste

**Directions:**
1. Cut the chicken breast into 6 fillets and season with a little salt and pepper.
2. Beat the egg in a bowl.
3. Pass the chicken breast in the egg and then in the grated cheese, sprinkling the fillets.
4. Non-stick and put in the air fryer at 400°F for about 30 minutes or until golden brown.

Cal 114 | Carb 13g | Fat 5.9g | Protein 2.3g | Sugar 3.2g

# Duck thighs

**Preparation Time:** 5 minutes | **Cooking Time:** 50 minutes | **Serves:** 4

**Ingredients:**
- 2pcs. Duck legs
- 1 tsp salt
- 1 tsp spice mixture (for ducks and geese)

- 1 tsp olive oil

**Directions:**
1. For the duck legs of the Air fryer the duck leg wash and pat dry. Mix the oil with the salt and the spice mixture and rub the duck legs around with it.
2. Place the spiced duck legs on the rack of the hot air fryer and cook at 390°F in 40 minutes. After 20 minutes, turn the legs once. Enjoy!

# Chicken Breast

**Preparation Time:** 30 minutes | **Cooking Time:** 25 minutes | **Serves:** 6

**Ingredients:**
- 1 lb. diced clean chicken breast
- ½ lemon
- Smoked paprika to taste
- Black pepper or chili powder, to taste
- Salt to taste

**Directions:**
1. Flavor the chicken with salt, paprika and pepper and marinate.
2. Store in Air fryer and turn on for 15 minutes at 350°F.
3. Turn the chicken over and raise the temperature to 390°F, and turn the Air Fryer on for another 5 minutes or until golden. Serve immediately.

Cal 124 | Carb 0g | Fat 1.4g | Protein 26.1g | Sugar 0g

# Spiced Chicken wings in Air fryer

**Preparation Time:** 15 minutes | **Cooking Time:** 30 minutes | **Serves:** 4

**Ingredients:**
- 1 kg chicken wings
- Salt
- Ground pepper
- Extra virgin olive oil
- Spices, I put roasted chicken or roast chicken spices.

**Directions:**
1. Clean the wings and chop, throw the tip and place in a bowl the other two parts of the wings that have more meat.
2. Season and add some extra virgin olive oil threads.
3. Sprinkle with spices
4. Flirt well and leave for 30 minutes to rest in the refrigerator.

5. Put the wings in the basket of the Air fryer and select 360°F, about 30 minutes. From 20 minutes, check if you have to remove them before.
6. From time to time, shake the basket so that the wings move and are made all over their faces. Serve and enjoy!

Cal 170 | Fat 6g | Carb 8g | Protein 15g

---

## Roasted Thigh

**Preparation Time:** 5 minutes | **Cooking Time:** 30 minutes | **Serves:** 1

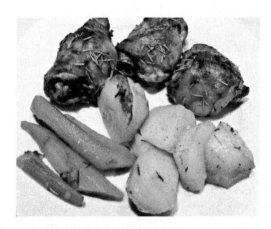

**Ingredients:**
- 3 chicken thighs and thighs
- 2 red seasonal bags
- 1 clove garlic
- ½ tsp of salt
- 1 pinch of black pepper

**Directions:**
1. Season chicken with red season, minced garlic, salt, and pepper. Leave to act for 5-10 minutes to obtain the flavor.
2. Put the chicken in the basket of the air fryer and bake at 390ºF for 20 minutes.
3. After that time, remove the Air Fryer basket and check the chicken spot. If it is still raw or not golden enough, turn it over and leave it for another 10 minutes at 350ºF.
4. After the previous step, your chicken will be ready on the Air Fryer! Serve with doré potatoes and leaf salad.

Cal 278 | Carb 0.1g | Fat 18g | Protein 31g

# Coxinha Fit

**Preparation Time:** 10 minutes | **Cooking Time:** 10-15 minutes | **Serves:** 4

**Ingredients:**
- ½ lb. seasoned and minced chicken
- 1 cup light cottage cheese
- 1 egg
- Condiments to taste
- Flaxseed or oatmeal

**Directions:**
1. In a bowl, mix all of the ingredients together except flour.
2. Knead well with your hands and mold into coxinha format.
3. If you prefer you can fill it, add chicken or cheese.
4. Repeat the process until all the dough is gone.
5. Pass the drumsticks in the flour and put them in the fryer.
6. Bake for 10 to 15 minutes at 390°F or until golden. Enjoy!

Cal 220 | Carb 40g | Fat 18g | Protein 100g | Sugar 5g

# Chicken in Beer

**Preparation Time:** 5 minutes | **Cooking Time:** 10 minutes | **Serves:** 4

**Ingredients:**
- 2 ¼ lbs chicken thigh and thigh
- ½ can of beer
- 4 cloves of garlic
- 1 large onion
- Pepper and salt to taste

**Directions:**
1. Wash the chicken pieces and, if desired, remove the skin to be healthier.
2. Place on an ovenproof plate.
3. In the blender, beat the other ingredients: beer, onion, garlic, and add salt and pepper, all together.
4. Cover the chicken with this mixture; it has to stay like swimming in the beer.
5. Take to the preheated air fryer at 390°F for 45 minutes.
6. It will roast when it has a brown cone on top and the beer has dried a bit.

Cal 674 | Carb 5.47g | Fat 41.94g | Protein 61.94g

# Rolled Turkey Breast

**Preparation Time:** 5 minutes | **Cooking Time:** 10 minutes | **Serves:** 4

**Ingredients:**
- 1 box of cherry tomatoes
- ¼ lb. turkey blanket

**Directions:**
1. Wrap the turkey and blanket in the tomatoes, close with the help of toothpicks.
2. Take to Air Fryer for 10 minutes at 390°F.
3. You can increase the filling with ricotta and other preferred light ingredients.

Cal 172 | Carb 3g | Fat 2g | Protein 34g | Sugar 1g

# Crispy Old Bay Chicken Wings

**Preparation Time:** 10 minutes | **Cooking Time:** 15 minutes | **Serves:** 4

**Ingredients:**
- Olive oil
- 2 tablespoons Old Bay seasoning
- 2 teaspoons baking powder
- 2 teaspoons salt
- 2 pounds chicken wings

**Directions:**
1. Spray a fryer basket lightly with olive oil.
2. In a big resealable bag, combine together the Old Bay seasoning, baking powder, and salt.
3. Pat the wings dry with paper towels.
4. Place the wings in the zip-top bag, seal, and toss with the seasoning mixture until evenly coated.
5. Place the seasoned wings in the fryer basket in a single layer. Lightly spray with olive oil.
6. Air fry for 7 minutes. Turn the wings over, lightly spray them with olive oil, and air fry until the wings are crispy and lightly browned, 5 to 8 more minutes. Using a meat thermometer, check to make sure the internal temperature is 165°F or higher.

Cal 501 | Fat 36g | Carb 1g | Protein 42g

# Chicken wings with Provencal herbs

**Preparation Time:** 15 minutes | **Cooking Time:** 20 minutes | **Serves:** 4

**Ingredients:**

- 1kg chicken wings
- Provencal herbs
- Extra virgin olive oil
- Salt
- Ground pepper

**Directions:**

1. Put the chicken wings in a bowl, clean and chopped.
2. Add a few threads of oil, salt, ground pepper and sprinkle with Provencal herbs.
3. Linked well and let macerate 15 minutes.
4. Take to the preheated air fryer at 360°F for 20 minutes.
5. From time to time, remove so that they are done on all their faces.
6. If see that they have been little golden, put a few more minutes.
7. Serve and enjoy!

Cal 160 | Fat 6g | Carb 8g| Protein 13g

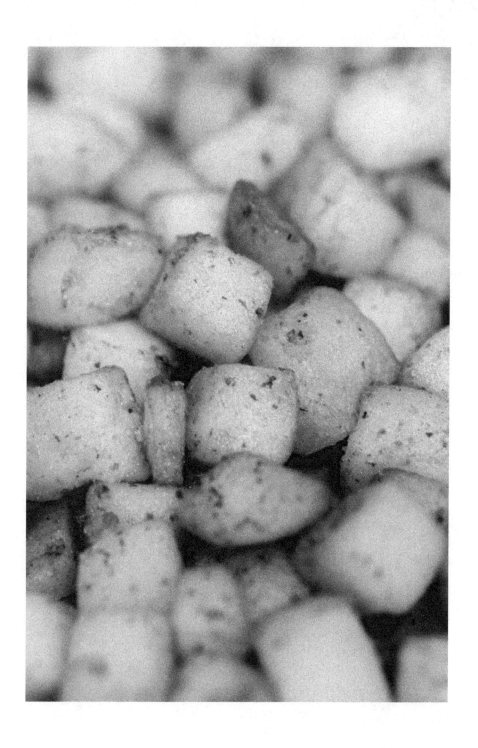

# Veggie Recipes

## Seasoned Yellow Squash

**Preparation Time:** 5 minutes | **Cooking Time:** 10 minutes | **Serves:** 4

**Ingredients:**
- Large yellow squash – 4, cut into slices
- Olive oil – ¼ cup
- Onion – ½, sliced
- Italian seasoning – ¾ tsp.
- Garlic salt – ½ tsp.
- Seasoned salt – ¼ tsp.

**Directions:**
1. In a bowl, mix all the ingredients together. Place the veggie mixture in the greased cooking tray.
2. Arrange the drip pan in the bottom of the Air Fryer Oven cooking chamber.
3. Take to the preheated air fryer at 400°F for 10 minutes.
4. Serve hot.

Cal 113 | Carb 8.1g | Fat 9g | Protein 4.2g

## Spicy Zucchini

**Preparation Time:** 10 minutes | **Cooking Time:** 15 minutes | **Serves:** 4

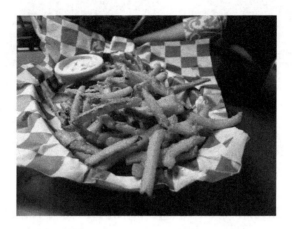

**Ingredients:**
- Zucchini – 1 lb. cut into ½-inch thick slices lengthwise
- Olive oil – 1 tbsp.
- Garlic powder – ½ tsp.
- Cayenne pepper – ½ tsp.
- Salt and ground black pepper, as required

**Directions:**
1. Put all of the ingredients into a bowl and toss to coat well.
2. Arrange the zucchini slices onto a cooking tray.
3. Arrange the drip pan in the bottom of the Air Fryer Oven cooking chamber.
4. Take to the preheated air fryer at 400°F for 12 minutes.
5. Serve hot.

Cal 67 | Carb 5.6g | Fat 5g | Protein 2g

---

## Buttered Asparagus

**Preparation Time:** 5 minutes | **Cooking Time:** 10 minutes | **Serves:** 4

**Ingredients:**
- Fresh thick asparagus spears – 1 lb. trimmed
- Butter – 1 tbsp. melted
- Salt and ground black pepper, as required

**Directions:**
1. Put all of the ingredients into a bowl and toss to coat well. Arrange the asparagus onto a cooking tray.
2. Arrange the drip pan in the bottom of the Air Fryer Oven cooking chamber.
3. Take to the preheated air fryer at 350°F for 10 minutes.

4. Serve hot.

Cal 64 | Carb 5.9g | Fat 4g | Protein 3.4g

---

# Garlic Thyme Mushrooms

**Preparation Time:** 5 minutes | **Cooking Time:** 10 minutes | **Serves:** 4

**Ingredients:**
- 3 tablespoons unsalted butter, melted
- 1 (8-ounce) package button mushrooms, sliced
- 2cloves garlic, minced
- 3sprigs fresh thyme leaves
- ½ teaspoon fine sea salt

**Directions:**
1. Preparing the Ingredients. Grease the basket with avocado oil. Preheat the air fryer to 400°F.
2. Place all the ingredients in a medium-sized bowl. Use a spoon or your hands to coat the mushroom slices.
3. Air Frying. Put the mushrooms in the basket in one layer; work in batches if necessary. Cook for 10 minutes, or until slightly crispy and brown. Garnish with thyme sprigs before serving.
4. Reheat in a warmed up 350°F air fryer for 5 minutes, or until heated through.

Cal 82 | Fat 9g | Protein 1g | Carb 1g | Fiber 0.2g

---

# Seasoned Carrots with Green Beans

**Preparation Time:** 5 minutes | **Cooking Time:** 10 minutes | **Serves:** 4

**Ingredients:**
- Green beans – ½ lb. trimmed
- Carrots – ½ lb. peeled and cut into sticks
- Olive oil – 1 tbsp.
- Salt and ground black pepper, as required

**Directions:**
1. Gather all the ingredients into a bowl and toss to coat well.
2. Place the vegetables in the rotisserie basket and attach the lid.
3. Arrange the drip pan in the bottom of the Air Fryer Oven cooking chamber. Take to the preheated air fryer at 400°F for 10 minutes.
4. Serve hot.

Cal 94 | Carb 12.7g | Fat 4.8g | Protein 2g

# Sweet Potato with Broccoli

**Preparation Time:** 5 minutes | **Cooking Time:** 20 minutes | **Serves:** 4

**Ingredients:**
- Medium sweet potatoes – 2, peeled and cut in 1-inch cubes
- Broccoli head – 1, cut in 1-inch florets
- Vegetable oil – 2 tbsps.
- Salt and ground black pepper, as required

**Directions:**
1. Grease a baking dish that will fit in the Air Fryer Oven.
2. Gather all of the ingredients into a bowl and toss to coat well. Place the veggie mixture into the prepared baking dish in a single layer.
3. Arrange the drip pan in the bottom of the Air Fryer Oven cooking chamber.
4. Take to the preheated air fryer at 415°F for 20 minutes.
5. Serve hot

Cal 170 | Carb 25.2g | Fat 7.1g | Protein 2.9g

# Seasoned Veggies

**Preparation Time:** 5 minutes | **Cooking Time:** 12 minutes | **Serves:** 4

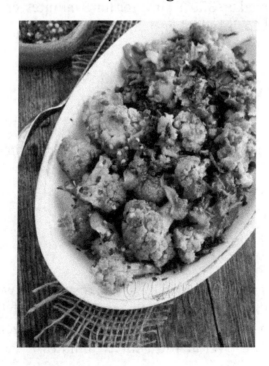

**Ingredients:**

- Baby carrots – 1 cup
- Broccoli florets – 1 cup
- Cauliflower florets – 1 cup
- Olive oil – 1 tbsp.
- Italian seasoning – 1 tbsp.
- Salt and ground black pepper, as required

**Directions:**

1. Gather all of the ingredients into a bowl and toss to coat well.
2. Place the vegetables in the rotisserie basket and attach the lid.
3. Arrange the drip pan in the bottom of the Air Fryer Oven cooking chamber.
4. Take to the preheated air fryer at 380°F for 18 minutes.
5. Serve

Cal 66 | Carb 5.7g | Fat 4.7g | Protein 1.4g

# Potato Gratin

**Preparation Time:** 5 minutes | **Cooking Time:** 20 minutes | **Serves:** 4

**Ingredients:**

- Large potatoes – 2, sliced thinly
- Cream – 5½ tbsps.
- Eggs – 2
- Plain flour – 1 tbsp.
- Cheddar cheese – ½ cup, grated

**Directions:**

1. Arrange the potato cubes onto the greased rack.
2. Arrange the drip pan in the bottom of the Air Fryer Oven cooking chamber. Take to the preheated air fryer at 355°F for 10 minutes
3. Meanwhile, in a bowl, add cream, eggs and flour and mix until a thick sauce form.
4. Once cooking is done, remove the tray from the Air Fryer Oven. Divide the potato slices into 4 lightly greased ramekins evenly and top with the egg mixture, followed by the cheese.
5. Arrange the ramekins on top of a cooking rack.
6. Take to your Kalorik Maxx Air Fryer at 390°F for 10 minutes.
7. Serve warm.

Cal 233 | Carb 31.g | Fat 8g | Protein 9.7g

# Buttered Broccoli

**Preparation Time:** 5 minutes | **Cooking Time:** 15 minutes | **Serves:** 4

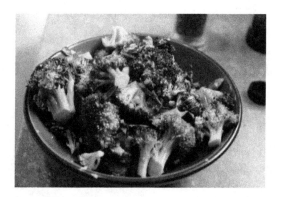

**Ingredients:**
- Broccoli florets – 1 lb.
- Butter – 1 tbsp. melted
- Red pepper flakes – ½ tsp. crushed
- Salt and ground black pepper, as required

**Directions:**
1. Gather all of the ingredients in a bowl and toss to coat well.
2. Place the broccoli florets in the rotisserie basket and attach the lid.
3. Arrange the drip pan in the bottom of the Air Fryer Oven cooking chamber.
4. Take to the preheated air fryer at 400°F for 15 minutes.
5. Serve immediately.

Cal 55 | Carb 6.1g | Fat 3g | Protein 2.3g

---

# Garlic Edamame

**Preparation Time:** 5 minutes | **Cooking Time:** 10 minutes | **Serves:** 4

**Ingredients:**
- Olive oil
- 1 (16-ounce) bag frozen edamame in pods
- salt and freshly ground black pepper
- ½ teaspoon garlic salt
- ½ teaspoon red pepper flakes (optional)

**Directions:**
1. Spray a fryer basket lightly with olive oil.

2. In a medium bowl, add the frozen edamame and lightly spray with olive oil. Toss to coat.
3. In a bowl, combine together the garlic salt, salt, black pepper, and red pepper flakes (if using). Add the mixture to the edamame and toss until evenly coated.
4. Place half the edamame in the fryer basket. Do not overfill the basket.
5. Air fry for 5 minutes. Shake the basket and cook until the edamame is starting to brown and get crispy, 3 to 5 more minutes.
6. Repeat with the remaining edamame and serve immediately.

Cal 100 | Fat 3g | Carb 9g | Protein 8g | Fiber 4g

## Pesto Gnocchi

**Preparation Time**: 5 minutes | **Cooking Time**: 15 minutes | **Serves**: 4

**Ingredients**:
- 1 tablespoon olive oil
- 1 onion, finely chopped
- cloves garlic, sliced
- 1 (16-ounce) package shelf-stable gnocchi
- 1 (8-ounce) jar pesto
- ⅓ cup grated Parmesan cheese

**Directions**:
1. Combine the oil, onion, garlic and gnocchi in a 6-by-6-by-2-inch pan. Put into your Kalorik Maxx Air Fryer.
2. Bake for 10 minutes, then remove the pan and stir.
3. Return the pan to the Air Fryer and cook for 5 to 10 minutes or until the gnocchi are lightly browned and crisp.
4. Remove the pan from the air fryer. Stir in the pesto and Parmesan cheese, and serve immediately.

Cal 646 | Fat 32g | Carb 69g | Fiber 2g | Protein 22g

## Spicy Chickpeas

**Preparation Time:** 5 minutes | **Cooking Time:** 20 minutes | **Serves:** 4

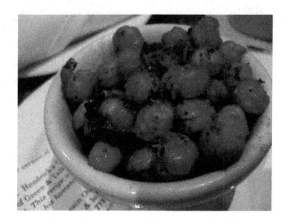

**Ingredients:**

- Olive oil
- ½ teaspoon ground cumin
- ½ teaspoon chili powder
- ¼ teaspoon cayenne pepper
- ¼ teaspoon salt
- 1 (19-ounce) can chickpeas, drained and rinsed

**Directions:**

1. Spray a fryer basket lightly with olive oil.
2. In a bowl, combine the chili powder, cumin, cayenne pepper, and salt.
3. In a medium bowl, add the chickpeas and lightly spray them with olive oil. Add the spice mixture and toss until coated evenly.
4. Transfer the chickpeas to the fryer basket. Air fry until the chickpeas reach your desired level of crunchiness, 15 to 20 minutes, making sure to shake the basket every 5 minutes.

Cal 122 |Fat 1g | Carb 22g | Protein 6g | Fiber 6g

# Crisp & Spicy Cabbage

**Preparation Time:** 5 Minutes | **Cooking Time:** 10 Minutes | **Serves:** 2

**Ingredients:**

- 1/2 Head White Cabbage, Chopped & Washed
- 1 Tablespoon Coconut Oil, Melted
- ¼ Teaspoon Cayenne Pepper
- ¼ Teaspoon Chili Powder
- ¼ Teaspoon Garlic Powder

**Directions:**

1. Turn on your air fryer to 390°F.

2. Mix your cabbage, spices and coconut oil together in a bowl, making sure your cabbage is coated well.
3. Place it in the fryer and cook for 10 minutes.

Cal 100 | Fat 2g | Carb 3g | Protein 5g

## Egg Roll Pizza Sticks

**Preparation Time:** 10 minutes | **Cooking Time:** 5 minutes | **Serves:** 4

**Ingredients:**
- Olive oil
- 8pieces reduced-fat string cheese
- 8egg roll wrappers
- 24slices turkey pepperoni
- Marinara sauce, for dipping (optional)

**Directions:**
1. Spray a fryer basket lightly with olive oil. Fill a small bowl with water.
2. Place each egg roll wrapper diagonally on a work surface. It should look like a diamond.
3. Place 3 slices of turkey pepperoni in a vertical line down the center of the wrapper.
4. Place 1 mozzarella cheese stick on top of the turkey pepperoni.
5. Fold the top and bottom corners of the egg roll wrapper over the cheese stick.
6. Fold the left corner over the cheese stick and roll the cheese stick up to resemble a spring roll. Dip a finger in the water and seal the edge of the roll
7. Repeat with the rest of the pizza sticks.
8. Place them in the fryer basket in a single layer, making sure to leave a little space between each one. Lightly spray the pizza sticks with oil.
9. Air fry until the pizza sticks are lightly browned and crispy, about 5 minutes.
10. These are best served hot while the cheese is melted. Accompany with a small bowl of marinara sauce, if desired.

Cal 362 | Fat 8g | Carb 40g | Protein 23g | Fiber 1g

## Cauliflower Rice

**Preparation Time:** 10 minutes | **Cooking Time:** 7 minutes | **Serves:** 4

**Ingredients:**
- 14 ounces cauliflower heads
- 1 tablespoon coconut oil
- 2 tablespoons fresh parsley, chopped

**Directions:**

1. Wash the cauliflower heads carefully and chop them into small pieces of rice.
2. Place the cauliflower in the air fryer and add coconut oil.
3. Stir carefully and cook for 5 minutes at 370° F.
4. Then add the fresh parsley and stir well.
5. Cook the cauliflower rice for 2 minutes more at 400° F.
6. After this, gently toss the cauliflower rice and serve immediately.

Cal 55 | Fat 3.5g | Fiber 2.5g | Carbs 5.4g | Protein 2g

## Balsamic Kale

**Preparation Time:** 2 minutes | **Cooking Time:** 12 minutes | **Serves:** 6

**Ingredients:**

- 2 tablespoons olive oil
- 3 garlic cloves, minced
- 2 and ½ pounds kale leaves
- Salt and black pepper to the taste
- 2 tablespoons balsamic vinegar

**Directions:**

1. In a pan that fits the air fryer, combine all the ingredients and toss.
2. Put the pan in your air fryer and cook at 300°F for 12 minutes.
3. Divide between plates and serve.

Cal 122 | Fat 4g | Fiber 3g | Carb 4g | Protein 5g

## Cajun Zucchini Chips

**Preparation Time:** 10 minutes | **Cooking Time:** 15 minutes | **Serves:** 4

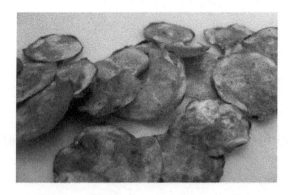

**Ingredients:**

- Olive oil
- 2 large zucchinis, cut into ⅛-inch-thick slices
- 2 teaspoons Cajun seasoning

**Directions:**

1. Spray a fryer basket lightly with olive oil.
2. Put the zucchini slices in a medium bowl and spray them generously with olive oil.
3. Sprinkle the Cajun seasoning over the zucchini and stir to make sure they are evenly coated with oil and seasoning.
4. Place slices in a single layer in the fryer basket, making sure not to overcrowd.
5. Air fry for 8 minutes. Flip the slices over and air fry until they are as crisp and brown as you prefer, an additional 7 to 8 minutes.

Cal 26 | Fat <1g | Carb 5g | Protein 2g | Fiber 2g

# Creamy Cabbage

**Preparation Time:** 10 minutes | **Cooking Time:** 20 minutes | **Serves:** 2

**Ingredients:**

- ½ green cabbage head, chopped
- ½ yellow onion, chopped
- Salt and black pepper, to taste
- ½ cup whipped cream
- 1 tablespoon cornstarch

**Directions:**

1. Put cabbage and onion in the air fryer.
2. In a bowl, mix cornstarch with cream, salt, and pepper. Stir and pour over cabbage.
3. Toss and cook at 400°F for 20 minutes.
4. Serve.

Cal 208 | Fat: 10g | Carb: 16g | Protein: 5g

# Cinnamon and Sugar Peaches

**Preparation Time:** 10 minutes | **Cooking Time:** 13 minutes | **Serves:** 4

**Ingredients:**

- Olive oil
- 2 tablespoons sugar
- ¼ teaspoon ground cinnamon

- 4 peaches, cut into wedges

**Directions:**
1. Spray a fryer basket lightly with olive oil.
2. In a bowl, combine the cinnamon and sugar. Add the peaches and toss to coat evenly.
3. Place the peaches in a single layer in the fryer basket on their sides.
4. Air fry for 5 minutes. Turn the peaches skin side down, lightly spray them with oil, and air fry until the peaches are lightly brown and caramelized, 5 to 8 more minutes.
5. Make it Even Lower Calorie: Use a zero-calorie sugar substitute such as NutraSweet or monk fruit sweetener instead of granulated sugar.

Cal 67 | Fat <1g | Carb 17g | Protein 1g | Fiber 2g

## Spicy Cabbage

**Preparation Time:** 5 minutes | **Cooking Time:** 7 minutes | **Serves:** 4

**Ingredients:**
- 1 head cabbage, sliced into 1-inch-thick ribbons
- 1 tablespoon olive oil
- 1 teaspoon garlic powder
- 1 teaspoon red pepper flakes
- 1 teaspoon salt
- 1 teaspoon freshly ground black pepper

**Directions:**
1. Toss the cabbage with the olive oil, garlic powder, red pepper flakes, salt, and pepper in a large mixing bowl until well coated.
2. Transfer the cabbage to the baking pan.
3. Slide the baking pan into Rack Position 1, select Convection Bake, set temperature to 350ºF and set time to 7 minutes.
4. Flip the cabbage with tongs halfway through the cooking time.
5. When cooking is complete, the cabbage should be crisp. Remove from the oven to a plate and serve warm.

Cal 172 | Fat 9.8g |Carb 17.5g | Protein 3.9g

## Spicy Broccoli with Hot Sauce

**Preparation Time:** 5 minutes | **Cooking Time:** 14 minutes | **Serves:** 6

**Ingredients:**

Broccoli:

- 1 medium-sized head broccoli, cut into florets
- 1½ tablespoons olive oil
- 1 teaspoon shallot powder
- 1 teaspoon porcini powder
- ½ teaspoon freshly grated lemon zest
- ½ teaspoon hot paprika
- ½ teaspoon granulated garlic
- ⅓ teaspoon fine sea salt
- ⅓ teaspoon celery seeds

Hot Sauce:

- ½ cup tomato sauce
- 1 tablespoon balsamic vinegar
- ½ teaspoon ground allspice

**Directions:**

1. In a mixing bowl, combine all the ingredients for the broccoli and toss to coat. Transfer the broccoli to your Kalorik Maxx Air Fryer basket.
2. Put in the air fryer basket and cook at 360°F for 14 minutes.
3. Meanwhile, make the hot sauce by whisking together the tomato sauce, balsamic vinegar, and allspice in a small bowl.
4. When cooking is complete, remove the broccoli from the oven and serve with the hot sauce.

Cal 191 | Fat 6g | Carb 31.4g |Protein 3.7g

# Cheesy Broccoli Gratin

**Preparation Time:** 5 minutes | **Cooking Time:** 14 minutes | **Serves:** 2

**Ingredients:**

- ⅓ cup fat-free milk
- 1 tablespoon all-purpose or gluten-free flour
- ½ tablespoon olive oil
- ½ teaspoon ground sage
- ¼ teaspoon kosher salt
- ⅛ teaspoon freshly ground black pepper
- 2 cups roughly chopped broccoli florets
- 6tablespoons shredded Cheddar cheese
- 2 tablespoons panko bread crumbs
- 1 tablespoon grated Parmesan cheese

- Olive oil spray

**Directions:**
1. Spritz the baking pan with olive oil spray.
2. Mix the milk, flour, olive oil, sage, salt, and pepper in a medium bowl and whisk to combine. Stir in the broccoli florets, Cheddar cheese, bread crumbs, and Parmesan cheese and toss to coat.
3. Pour the broccoli mixture into the prepared baking pan.
4. Select Convection Bake set temperature to 330ºF and set time to 14 minutes.
5. When cooking is complete, the top should be golden brown and the broccoli should be tender. Remove from the oven and serve immediately.

Cal 172 | Fat 9.8g | Carb 17.5g | Protein 3.9g

## Coconut Oil Artichokes

**Preparation Time:** 10 minutes | **Cooking Time:** 8 minutes | **Serves:** 4

**Ingredients:**
- 1-pound artichokes
- 1 tablespoon coconut oil
- 1 tablespoon water
- ½ teaspoon minced garlic
- ¼ teaspoon cayenne pepper

**Directions:**
1. Trim the ends of the artichokes, sprinkle them with the water, and rub them with the minced garlic.
2. Sprinkle with the cayenne pepper and the coconut oil.
3. After this, wrap the artichokes in foil and place in the air fryer basket.
4. Cook for 5 minutes at 370° F.
5. Then remove the artichokes from the foil and cook them for 3 minutes more at 400° F.
6. Transfer the cooked artichokes to serving plates and allow to cool a little. Serve.

Cal 83 | Fat 3.6g |Fiber 6.2g | Carbs 12.1g | Protein 3.7g

## Rosti (Swiss potatoes)

**Preparation Time:** 10 minutes | **Cooking Time:** 15 minutes | **Serves:** 4

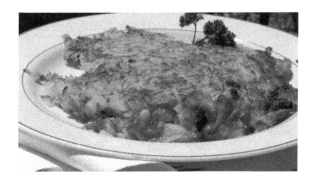

**Ingredients:**
- 250 g peeled white potatoes
- 1 tablespoon finely chopped chives
- Freshly ground black pepper
- 1 tablespoon of olive oil
- 2 tablespoons of sour cream

**Directions:**
1. Preheat the air fryer to 360°F. Grate the thick potatoes in a bowl and add three quarters of the chives and salt and pepper to taste. Mix it well.
2. Grease the pizza pan with olive oil and spread the potato mixture evenly through the pan. Press the grated potatoes against the pan and spread the top of the potato cake with some olive oil.
3. Place the pizza pan inside the fryer basket and insert it into your Kalorik Maxx Air Fryer. Set the timer to 15 mins and fry the rosti until it has a nice brownish color on the outside and is soft and well done inside.
4. Cut the rosti into 4 quarters and place each quarter on a plate. Garnish with a spoonful of sour cream. Spread the remaining of the scallions over the sour cream and add a touch of ground pepper.

# Zucchini Curry

**Preparation Time:** 5 Minutes | **Cooking Time:** 8-10 Minutes | **Serves:** 2

**Ingredients:**
- 2 Zucchinis, Washed & Sliced
- 1 Tablespoon Olive Oil
- Pinch Sea Salt
- Curry Mix, Pre-Made

**Directions:**
1. Turn on your air fryer to 390°F.
2. Combine your zucchini slices, salt, oil, and spices.

3. Put the zucchini into your Kalorik Maxx Air Fryer, cooking for eight to ten minutes.
4. You can serve alone or with sour cream.

Cal 100 | Fat 1g | Carb 4g | Protein 2g

## Veggies on Toast

**Preparation Time**: 12 minutes | **Cooking Time**: 10 minutes | **Serves**: 4

**Ingredients**:
- 1 red bell pepper, cut into ½-inch strips
- 1 cup sliced button or cremini mushrooms
- 1 small yellow squash, sliced
- green onions, cut into ½-inch slices
- Extra light olive oil for misting
- to 6 pieces sliced French or Italian bread
- tablespoons softened butter
- ½ cup soft goat cheese

**Directions**:
1. Combine the red pepper, mushrooms, squash, and green onions in the air fryer and mist with oil. Roast for 5 to 9 minutes or until the vegetables are tender, shaking the basket once during cooking time.
2. Remove the vegetables from the basket and set aside.
3. Spread the bread with butter and place in the air fryer, butter-side up. Toast for 2 to 4 minutes or until golden brown.
4. Spread the goat cheese on the toasted bread and top with the vegetables; serve warm.
5. Variation tip: To add even more flavor, drizzle the finished toasts with extra-virgin olive oil and balsamic vinegar.

Cal 162 | Fat 11g | Carb 9g | Fiber 2g | Protein 7g

## Jumbo Stuffed Mushrooms

**Preparation Time**: 10 minutes | **Cooking Time**: 8 minutes | **Serves**: 4

**Ingredients**:
- jumbo portobello mushrooms
- 1 tablespoon olive oil
- ¼ cup ricotta cheese
- tablespoons Parmesan cheese, divided
- 1 cup frozen chopped spinach, thawed and drained

- ⅓ cup bread crumbs
- ¼ teaspoon minced fresh rosemary

**Directions**:

1. Wipe the mushrooms with a damp cloth. Remove the stems and discard. Using a spoon, gently scrape out most of the gills.
2. Rub the mushrooms with the olive oil. Put in the air fryer basket, hollow side up, and bake for 3 minutes. Carefully remove the mushroom caps, because they will contain liquid. Drain the liquid out of the caps.
3. In a medium bowl, combine the ricotta, 3 tablespoons of Parmesan cheese, spinach, bread crumbs, and rosemary, and mix well.
4. Stuff this mixture into the drained mushroom caps. Sprinkle with the remaining 2 tablespoons of Parmesan cheese. Put the mushroom caps back into the basket.
5. Bake for 4 to 6 minutes or until the filling is hot and the mushroom caps are tender.

Cal 117 | Fat 7g | Carb 8g | Fiber 1g | Protein 7g

## Healthy Carrot Fries

**Preparation Time:** 5 Minutes | **Cooking Time:** 12-15 Minutes| **Serves:** 2

**Ingredients:**

- 5 Large Carrots
- 1 Tablespoon Olive Oil
- ½ Teaspoon Sea Salt

**Directions:**

1. Heat your air fryer to 390°F, and then wash and peel your carrots. Cut them in a way to form fries.
2. Combine your carrot sticks with your olive oil and salt, coating evenly.
3. Place them into your Kalorik Maxx Air Fryer, cooking for twelve minutes. If they're not as crispy as you desire, then cook for two to three more minutes.
4. Serve with sour cream, ketchup or just with your favorite main dish.

Cal 140 | Fat 3g | Carb 6g | Protein 7g

## Simple Roasted Carrots

**Preparation Time:** 5 Minutes | **Cooking Time:** 35 Minutes

**Ingredients:**

- 4 Cups Carrots, Chopped
- 1 Teaspoon Herbs de Provence
- 2 Teaspoons Olive Oil

- 4 Tablespoons Orange Juice

**Directions:**
1. Start by preheating your air fryer to 320°F.
2. Combine your carrot pieces with your herbs and oil.
3. Cook for twenty-five to twenty-eight minutes.
4. Take it out and dip the pieces in orange juice before frying for an additional seven minutes.

Cal 125 | Fat 2g | Carb 5g | Protein 6g

---

# Broccoli & Cheese

**Preparation Time:** 5 Minutes | **Cooking Time:** 9 Minutes

**Ingredients:**
- 1 Head Broccoli, Washed & Chopped
- Salt & Pepper to Taste
- 1 Tablespoon Olive oil
- Sharp Cheddar Cheese, Shredded

**Directions:**
1. Start by putting your air fryer to 360°F.
2. Combine your broccoli with your olive oil and sea salt.
3. Place it in the air fryer, and cook for six minutes.
4. Take it out, and then top with cheese, cooking for another three minutes.
5. Serve with your choice of protein.

Cal 170 | Fat 5g | Carb 9g | Protein 7g

---

# Parmesan Asparagus Fries

**Preparation Time:** 15 minutes | **Cooking Time:** 6 minutes | **Serves:** 4

**Ingredients:**
- 2egg whites
- ¼ cup water
- ¼ cup plus 2 tablespoons grated Parmesan cheese, divided
- ¾ cup panko bread crumbs
- ¼ teaspoon salt
- 12 ounces (340 g) fresh asparagus spears, woody ends trimmed
- Cooking spray

**Directions:**

1. In a shallow dish, whisk together the egg whites and water until slightly foamy. In a separate shallow dish, thoroughly combine ¼ cup of Parmesan cheese, bread crumbs, and salt.
2. Dip the asparagus in the egg white, then roll in the cheese mixture to coat well.
3. Place the asparagus in the air fryer basket in a single layer, leaving space between each spear. Spritz the asparagus with cooking spray.
4. Put in the air fryer and cook at 390°F for 6 minutes.
5. When cooking is complete, the asparagus should be golden brown and crisp. Remove from the oven. Sprinkle with the remaining 2 tablespoons of cheese and serve hot.

Cal 191 | Fat 6g | Carb 31.4g | Protein 3.7g

## Cauliflower Hash

**Preparation Time:** 10 minutes | **Cooking Time:** 15 minutes |**Serves:** 6

**Ingredients:**
- 1-pound cauliflower
- 2 eggs
- 1 teaspoon salt
- ½ teaspoon ground paprika
- 4-ounce turkey fillet, chopped

**Directions:**
1. Wash the cauliflower, chop, and set aside.
2. In a different bowl, crack the eggs and whisk well.
3. Add the salt and ground paprika; stir.
4. Place the chopped turkey in the air fryer basket and cook it for 4 minutes at 365° F, stirring halfway through.
5. After this, add the chopped cauliflower and stir the mixture.
6. Cook the turkey/cauliflower mixture for 6 minutes more at 370° F, stirring it halfway through.
7. Then pour in the whisked egg mixture and stir it carefully.
8. Cook the cauliflower hash for 5 minutes more at 365° F.
9. When the cauliflower hash is done, let it cool and transfer to serving bowls. Serve and enjoy.

Cal 143 | Fat 9.5g | Fiber 2g| Carb 4.5g | Protein 10.4g

## Sweet Potato & Onion Mix

**Preparation Time:** 10 minutes | **Cooking Time:** 10 minutes | **Serves:** 4

**Ingredients:**

- 2 sweet potatoes, peeled
- 1 red onion, peeled
- 1 white onion, peeled
- 1 teaspoon olive oil
- ¼ cup almond milk

**Directions:**

1. Chop the sweet potatoes and the onions into cubes.
2. Sprinkle the sweet potatoes with olive oil.
3. Place the sweet potatoes in the air fryer basket and cook for 5 minutes at 400° F.
4. Then stir the sweet potatoes and add the chopped onions.
5. Pour in the almond milk and stir gently.
6. Cook the mix for 5 minutes more at 400° F.
7. When the mix is cooked, let it cool a little and serve.

Cal 56 | Fat 4.8g | Fiber 0.9g | Carbs 3.5g | Protein 0.6g

# Air Fried Roasted Corn on The Cob

**Preparation Time:** 5 minutes | **Cooking Time:** 10 minutes | **Serves:** 4

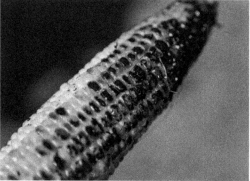

**Ingredients:**

- 1 tablespoon vegetable oil
- 4 ears of corn
- Unsalted butter, for topping
- Salt, for topping
- Freshly ground black pepper, for topping

**Directions:**

1. Preparing the Ingredients. Rub the vegetable oil onto the corn, coating it thoroughly.

2. Set the temperature to 400°F. Set the timer and grill for 5 minutes.
3. Using tongs, flip or rotate the corn.
4. Reset the timer and grill for 5 minutes more.
5. Serve with a pat of butter and a generous sprinkle of salt and pepper.

Cal 265 | Fat 17g | Carb 29g | Fiber 4g | Sugar 5g | Protein 5g

## Chili Broccoli

**Preparation Time:** 5 minutes | **Cooking Time:** 15 minutes | **Serves:** 4

**Ingredients:**
- 1-pound broccoli florets
- 2 tablespoons olive oil
- 2 tablespoons chili sauce
- Juice of 1 lime
- A pinch of salt and black pepper

**Directions:**
1. Combine all of the ingredients in a bowl, and toss well.
2. Put the broccoli in your air fryer's basket and cook at 400°F for 15 minutes.
3. Divide between plates and serve.

Cal 173 | Fat 6g | Fiber 2g | Carb 6g | Protein 8g

## Air Fried Honey Roasted Carrots

**Preparation Time:** 5 minutes | **Cooking Time:** 15 minutes | **Serves:** 4

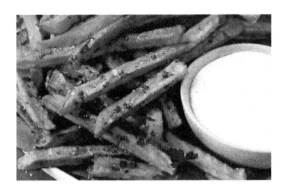

**Ingredients:**
- 3 cups baby carrots
- 1 tablespoon extra-virgin olive oil

- 1 tablespoon honey
- Salt
- Freshly ground black pepper
- Fresh dill (optional)

**Directions:**

1. Preparing the Ingredients. In a bowl, combine honey, olive oil, carrots, salt, and pepper. Make sure that the carrots are thoroughly coated with oil. Place the carrots in the air fryer basket.
2. Set the temperature to 390°F. Set the timer and roast for 12 minutes, or until fork-tender.
3. Remove the air fryer drawer and release the air fryer basket. Pour the carrots into a bowl, sprinkle with dill, if desired, and serve.

Cal 140 | Fat 3g | Carb 7g | Protein 9g

# Air Fried Roasted Cabbage

**Preparation Time:** 5 minutes | **Cooking Time:** 10 minutes | **Serves:** 4

**Ingredients:**

- 1 head cabbage, sliced in 1-inch-thick ribbons
- 1 tablespoon olive oil
- salt and freshly ground black pepper
- 1 teaspoon garlic powder
- 1 teaspoon red pepper flakes

**Directions**

1. Preparing the Ingredients. In a bowl, combine the olive oil, cabbage, salt, pepper, garlic powder, and red pepper flakes. Make sure that the cabbage is thoroughly coated with oil. Place the cabbage in the air fryer basket.
2. Set the temperature of your Air Fryer to 350°F. Set the timer and roast for 4 minutes.
3. Using tongs, flip the cabbage. Reset the timer and roast for 3 minutes more.

Cal 100 | Fat 1g | Carb 3g| Protein 3g

# Caramelized Broccoli

**Preparation Time:** 5 minutes | **Cooking Time:** 10 minutes | **Serves:** 4

**Ingredients:**

- 4 cups broccoli florets
- 3 tablespoons melted ghee or butter-flavored coconut oil
- 1½ teaspoons fine sea salt or smoked salt

- Mayonnaise, for serving (optional; omit for egg-free)

**Directions**

1. Preparing the Ingredients. Grease the basket with avocado oil. Preheat the air fryer to 400°F. Place the broccoli in a large bowl. Drizzle it with the ghee, toss to coat, and sprinkle it with the salt.
2. Air Frying. Transfer the broccoli to your Kalorik Maxx Air Fryer basket and cook for 8 minutes, or until tender and crisp on the edges.

Cal 120 | Fat 2g | Carb 4g | Protein 3g

## Brussels Sprouts with Balsamic Oil

**Preparation Time:** 5 minutes | **Cooking Time:** 15 minutes | **Serves:** 4

**Ingredients:**

- ¼ teaspoon salt
- 1 tablespoon balsamic vinegar
- 2 cups Brussels sprouts, halved
- 3 tablespoons olive oil

**Directions:**

1. Preparing the Ingredients. Preheat the air fryer for 5 minutes. Mix all ingredients in a bowl until the zucchini fries are well coated.
2. Air Frying. Place in the air fryer basket. Close and cook for 15 minutes for 350°F.

Cal 82 | Fat 6.8g | Protein 1.5g

## Shredded Cabbage

**Preparation Time:** 10 minutes | **Cooking Time:** 15 minutes | **Serves:** 4

**Ingredients:**

- 15 ounces cabbage
- ¼ teaspoon salt
- ¼ cup chicken stock
- ½ teaspoon paprika

**Directions:**

1. Shred the cabbage and sprinkle it with the salt and paprika.
2. Stir the cabbage and let it sit for 10 minutes.
3. Then transfer the cabbage to your Kalorik Maxx Air Fryer basket and add the chicken stock.
4. Cook the cabbage for 5 minutes at 250° F, stirring halfway through.

5. When the cabbage is soft, it is done.
6. Serve immediately, while still hot

Cal 132 | Fat 2.1g | Carbs 32.1g | Protein: 1.78g

---

# Charred Green Beans with Seeds

**Preparation Time:** 5 minutes | **Cooking Time:** 8 minutes | **Serves:** 4

**Ingredients:**
- 1 tablespoon reduced-sodium soy sauce or tamari
- ½ tablespoon Sriracha sauce
- 4teaspoons toasted sesame oil, divided
- 12 ounces (340 g) trimmed green beans
- ½ tablespoon toasted sesame seeds

**Directions:**
1. Whisk together the soy sauce, Sriracha sauce, and 1 teaspoon of sesame oil in a small bowl until smooth. Set aside.
2. Toss the green beans with the remaining sesame oil in a large bowl until evenly coated.
3. Place the green beans in the air fryer basket in a single layer.
4. Put the air fryer basket, set temperature to 375ºF and set time to 8 minutes.
5. Stir the green beans halfway through the cooking time.
6. When cooking is complete, the green beans should be lightly charred and tender. Remove from the oven to a platter. Pour the prepared sauce over the top of green beans and toss well. Serve sprinkled with the toasted sesame seeds.

Cal 191 | Fat 6g | Carb 31.4g | Protein 3.7g

# Fish & Seafood

## Cheesy Lemon Halibut

**Preparation Time:** 5 minutes | **Cooking Time:** 10 minutes | **Serves:** 4

**Ingredients:**
- 1 lb. halibut fillet
- ½ cup butter
- 2 ½ tbsp. mayonnaise
- 2 ½ tbsp. lemon juice
- ¾ cup parmesan cheese, grated

**Directions:**
1. Pre-heat your fryer at 375°F.
2. Spritz the halibut fillets with cooking spray and season as desired.
3. Put the halibut in the fryer and cook for twelve minutes.
4. In the meantime, combine the butter, mayonnaise, and lemon juice in a bowl with a hand mixer. Ensure a creamy texture is achieved.
5. Stir in the grated parmesan.
6. When the halibut is ready, open the drawer and spread the butter over the fish with a butter knife. Let it cook for a couple more minutes, then serve hot.

Cal 354 | Fat 21g | Carb 23g | Protein 19g

## Shrimp Croquettes

**Preparation Time**: 12 minutes | **Cooking Time**: 6 minutes | **Serves**: 3-4

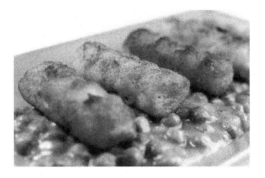

**Ingredients**:

- ⅔ pound cooked shrimp, shelled and deveined
- 1½ cups bread crumbs, divided
- 1 egg, beaten
- tablespoon lemon juice
- green onions, finely chopped
- ½ teaspoon dried basil
- Pinch salt
- Freshly ground black pepper
- tablespoons olive oil

**Directions**:

1. Finely chop the shrimp. Take about 1 tablespoon of the finely chopped shrimp and chop it further until it's almost a paste. Set aside.
2. In a medium bowl, combine ½ cup of the bread crumbs with the egg and lemon juice. Let stand for 5 minutes.
3. Stir the shrimp, green onions, basil, salt, and pepper into the bread crumb mixture.
4. Combine the remaining 1 cup of bread crumbs with the olive oil on a shallow plate; mix well.
5. Form the shrimp mixture into 1½-inch round balls and press firmly with your hands. Roll in the bread crumb mixture to coat.
6. Air-fry the little croquettes in batches for 6 to 8 minutes or until they are brown and crisp. Serve with cocktail sauce for dipping, if desired.

Cal 330 | Fat 12g | Carb 31g | Fiber 2g | Protein 24g

## Spicy Mackerel

**Preparation Time:** 5 minutes | **Cooking Time:** 10 minutes | **Serves:** 4

**Ingredients**:

- 2 mackerel fillets
- 2 tbsp. red chili flakes
- 2 tsp. garlic, minced
- 1 tsp. lemon juice

**Directions**:

1. Season the mackerel fillets with the red pepper flakes, minced garlic, and a drizzle of lemon juice. Allow to sit for five minutes.
2. Preheat your fryer at 350°F.
3. Cook the mackerel for five minutes, before opening the drawer, flipping the fillets, and allowing to cook on the other side for another five minutes.

4. Plate the fillets, making sure to spoon any remaining juice over them before serving.

Cal 393 | Fat 12g | Carb 13g | Protein 35g

---

# Thyme Scallops

**Preparation Time:** 5 minutes | **Cooking Time:** 10 minutes | **Serves:** 4

**Ingredients:**
- 1 lb. scallops
- Salt and pepper
- ½ tbsp. butter
- ½ cup thyme, chopped

**Directions:**
1. Wash the scallops and dry them completely. Season with pepper and salt, then set aside while you prepare the pan.
2. Grease a foil pan in several spots with the butter and cover the bottom with the thyme. Place the scallops on top.
3. Pre-heat the fryer at 400°F and set the rack inside.
4. Place the foil pan on the rack and allow to cook for seven minutes.
5. Take care when removing the pan from the fryer and transfer the scallops to a serving dish. Spoon any remaining butter in the pan over the fish and enjoy.

Cal 454 | Fat 18g | Carb 27g | Protein 34g

---

# Buttery Shrimp Skewers

**Preparation Time:** 5 minutes | **Cooking Time:** 10 minutes | **Serves:** 4

**Ingredients:**
- 8 shrimps; peeled and deveined
- 8 green bell pepper slices
- 1 tbsp. butter; melted
- 4 garlic cloves; minced
- Salt and black pepper to the taste

**Directions:**
1. In a bowl mix shrimp with garlic, butter, salt, pepper and bell pepper slices; toss to coat and leave aside for 10 minutes.
2. Arrange 2 shrimp and 2 bell pepper slices on a skewer and repeat with the rest of the shrimp and bell pepper pieces.
3. Place them all in your air fryer's basket and cook at 360°F, for 6 minutes. Divide among plates and serve right away.

Cal 140 | Fat 1g | Fiber 12g | Carb 15g | Protein 7g

## Mustard Salmon

**Preparation Time:** 5 minutes | **Cooking Time:** 10 minutes | **Serves:** 4

**Ingredients:**

- 1 big salmon fillet; boneless
- 2 tbsp. mustard
- 1 tbsp. coconut oil
- 1 tbsp. maple extract
- Salt and black pepper to the taste

**Directions:**

1. In a bowl mix maple extract with mustard, whisk well, season salmon with salt and pepper and brush salmon with this mix.
2. Spray some cooking spray over fish; place in your air fryer and cook at 370°F, for 10 minutes; flipping halfway. Serve with a tasty side salad.

Cal 300 | Fat 7g | Fiber 14g | Carb 16g | Protein 20g

## Chinese Style Cod

**Preparation Time:** 5 minutes | **Cooking Time:** 10 minutes | **Serves:** 2

**Ingredients:**

- 2 medium cod fillets; boneless
- 1 tbsp. light soy sauce
- 1/2 tsp. ginger; grated
- 1 tsp. peanuts; crushed
- 2 tsp. garlic powder

**Directions:**

1. Put fish fillets in a heat proof dish that fits your air fryer, add garlic powder, soy sauce and ginger; toss well, put in your air fryer and cook at 350°F, for 10 minutes.
2. Divide fish on plates, sprinkle peanuts on top and serve.

Cal 254 | Fat 10g | Fiber 11g | Carb 14g | Protein 23g

## Salmon and Orange Marmalade

**Preparation Time:** 5 minutes | **Cooking Time:** 20 minutes | **Serves:** 4

**Ingredients:**

- 1 lb. wild salmon; skinless, boneless and cubed
- 1/4 cup orange juice
- 1/3 cup orange marmalade
- 1/4 cup balsamic vinegar
- A pinch of salt and black pepper

**Directions:**
1. Heat up a pot with the vinegar over medium heat; add marmalade and orange juice; stir, bring to a simmer, cook for 1 minute and take off heat.
2. Thread salmon cubes on skewers, season with salt and black pepper, brush them with half of the orange marmalade mix, arrange in your air fryer's basket and cook at 360°F, for 3 minutes on each side. Brush skewers with the rest of the vinegar mix; divide among plates and serve right away with a side salad.

Cal 240 | Fat 9g | Fiber 12g | Carb 14g | Protein 10g

# Tilapia & Chives Sauce

**Preparation Time:** 5 minutes | **Cooking Time:** 10 minutes | **Serves:** 4

**Ingredients:**
- 4 medium tilapia fillets
- 2 tsp. honey
- Juice from 1 lemon
- 2 tbsp. chives; chopped
- Salt and black pepper to the taste

**Directions:**
1. Flavor fish with salt and pepper, spray with cooking spray, place in preheated air fryer 350°F and cook for 8 minutes; flipping halfway.
2. Meanwhile in a bowl, mix honey, salt, pepper, chives and lemon juice and whisk really well. Divide air fryer fish on plates, drizzle yogurt sauce all over and serve right away.

Cal 261 | Fat 8g | Fiber 18g | Carb 24g | Protein 21g

# Marinated Salmon Recipe

**Preparation Time:** 65 minutes | **Cooking Time:** 30 minutes | **Serves:** 4

**Ingredients:**
- 1 whole salmon
- 1 tbsp. tarragon; chopped
- 1 tbsp. garlic; minced
- Juice from 2 lemons

- A pinch of salt and black pepper

**Directions:**
1. In a large fish, mix fish with salt, pepper and lemon juice; toss well and keep in the fridge for 1 hour.
2. Stuff salmon with garlic and place in your air fryer's basket and cook at 320°F, for 25 minutes. Divide among plates and serve with a tasty coleslaw on the side.

Cal 300 | Fat 8g | Fiber 9g | Carb 19g | Protein 27g

## Tasty Grilled Red Mullet

**Preparation Time:** 5 minutes | **Cooking Time:** 10 minutes | **Serves:** 8

**Ingredients:**
- 8 whole red mullets, gutted and scales removed
- Salt and pepper to taste
- Juice from 1 lemon
- 1 tablespoon olive oil

**Directions:**
1. Preheat the air fryer at 390°F.
2. Place the grill pan attachment in the air fryer.
3. Season the red mullet with salt, pepper, and lemon juice.
4. Brush with olive oil.
5. Grill for 15 minutes.

Cal 152 | Carb 0.9g | Protein 23.1g | Fat 6.2g

## Cajun Salmon

**Preparation Time:** 5 minutes | **Cooking Time:** 10 minutes | **Serves:** 2

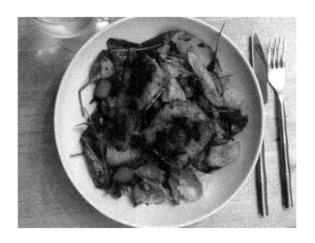

**Ingredients:**
- Salmon fillet (1 - 7 oz.) 0.75-inches thick
- Cajun seasoning
- Juice (¼ of a lemon)
- Optional: Sprinkle of sugar

**Directions:**
1. Set the Air Fryer at 356º F to preheat for five minutes.
2. Rinse and dry the salmon with a paper towel. Cover the fish with the Cajun coating mix.
3. Place the fillet in the air fryer for seven minutes with the skin side up.
4. Serve with a sprinkle of lemon and dusting of sugar if desired.

Cal 285 | Fat 17.8g | Carb 6.8g | Protein 42.1g

## Garlicky-Grilled Turbot

**Preparation Time:** 5 minutes | **Cooking Time:** 20 minutes | **Serves:** 2

**Ingredients:**
- 2 whole turbot, scaled and head removed
- Salt and pepper to taste
- 1 clove of garlic, minced
- ½ cup chopped celery leaves
- 2 tablespoons olive oil

**Directions:**
1. Preheat the air fryer at 390°F.
2. Place the grill pan attachment in the air fryer.
3. Flavor the turbot with salt, pepper, garlic, and celery leaves.
4. Brush with oil.

5. Cook in the grill pan for 20 minutes until the fish becomes flaky.

Cal 269 | Carb 3.3g | Protein 66.2g | Fat 25.6g

---

## Char-Grilled Spicy Halibut

**Preparation Time:** 5 minutes | **Cooking Time:** 20 minutes | **Serves:** 4

**Ingredients:**
- 3 pounds halibut fillet, skin removed
- Salt and pepper to taste
- 4 tablespoons olive oil
- 2 cloves of garlic, minced
- 1 tablespoon chili powder

**Directions:**
1. Place all ingredients in a Ziploc bag.
2. Keep it in the fridge for at least 2 hours.
3. Preheat the air fryer at 390°F. Place the grill pan attachment in the air fryer.
4. Grill the fish for 20 minutes while flipping every 5 minutes.

Cal 385 | Carb 1.7g | Protein 33g | Fat 40.6g

---

## Swordfish with Charred Leeks

**Preparation Time:** 5 minutes | **Cooking Time:** 20 minutes | **Serves:** 4

**Ingredients:**
- 4 swordfish steaks
- Salt and pepper to taste
- 3 tablespoons lime juice
- 2 tablespoons olive oil
- 4 medium leeks, cut into an inch long

**Directions:**
1. Preheat the air fryer at 390°F.
2. Place the grill pan attachment in the air fryer.
3. Season the swordfish with salt, pepper and lime juice.
4. Brush the fish with olive oil. Place fish fillets on grill pan and top with leeks.
5. Grill for 20 minutes.

Cal 611 | Carb 14.6g | Protein 48g | Fat 40g

# Breaded Coconut Shrimp

**Preparation Time:** 5 minutes | **Cooking Time:** 15 minutes | **Serves:** 4

**Ingredients:**
- Shrimp (1 lb.)
- Panko breadcrumbs (1 cup)
- Shredded coconut (1 cup)
- Eggs (2)
- All-purpose flour (.33 cup)

**Directions:**
1. Fix the temperature of the Air Fryer at 360ºF.
2. Peel and devein the shrimp.
3. Whisk the seasonings with the flour as desired. In another dish, whisk the eggs, and in the third container, combine the breadcrumbs and coconut.
4. Dip the cleaned shrimp into the flour, egg wash, and finish it off with the coconut mixture.
5. Lightly spray the basket of the fryer and set the timer for 10-15 minutes.
6. Air-fry until it's a golden brown before serving.

Cal 285 | Fat 12.8g | Carb 3.7g | Protein 38.1g

# Cod Fish Nuggets

**Preparation Time:** 5 minutes | **Cooking Time:** 20 minutes | **Serves:** 4

**Ingredients:**
- Cod fillet (1 lb.)
- Eggs (3)
- Olive oil (4 tbsp.)
- Almond flour (1 cup)
- Gluten-free breadcrumbs (1 cup)

**Directions:**
1. Warm the Air Fryer at 390º F.
2. Slice the cod into nuggets.
3. Prepare three bowls. Whisk the eggs in one. Combine the salt, oil, and breadcrumbs in another. Sift the almond flour into the third one.
4. Cover each of the nuggets with the flour, dip in the eggs, and the breadcrumbs.
5. Arrange the nuggets in the basket and set the timer for 20 minutes.
6. Serve the fish with your favorite dips or sides.

Cal 334 | Fat 10g | Carb 8g | Protein 32g

# Grilled Sardines

**Preparation Time:** 5 minutes | **Cooking Time:** 20 minutes | **Serves:** 4

**Ingredients:**
- 5 sardines
- Herbs of Provence

**Direction:**
1. Preheat the air fryer to 320°F.
2. Spray the basket and place your sardines in the basket of your fryer.
3. Set the timer for 14 minutes. After 7 minutes, remember to turn the sardines so that they are roasted on both sides.

Cal 189g | Fat 10g | Carb 0g | Sugars 0g | Protein 22g

---

# Fried Catfish

**Preparation Time:** 5 minutes | **Cooking Time:** 15 minutes | **Serves:** 4

**Ingredients:**
- Olive oil (1 tbsp.)
- Seasoned fish fry (.25 cup)
- Catfish fillets (4)

**Directions:**
1. Heat the Air Fryer to reach 400º F before fry time.
2. Rinse the catfish and pat dry using a paper towel.
3. Dump the seasoning into a sizeable zipper-type bag. Add the fish and shake to cover each fillet. Spray with a spritz of cooking oil spray and add to the basket.
4. Set the timer for 10 minutes. Flip, and reset the timer for ten additional minutes. Turn the fish once more and cook for 2-3 minutes.
5. Once it reaches the desired crispiness, transfer to a plate, and serve.

Cal 376 | Fat 9g | Carb 10g | Protein 28g

---

# Creamy Salmon

**Preparation Time:** 5 minutes | **Cooking Time:** 20 minutes | **Serves:** 4

**Ingredients:**
- Chopped dill (1 tbsp.)
- Olive oil (1 tbsp.)
- Sour cream (3 tbsp.)
- Plain yogurt (1.76 oz.)
- Salmon (6 pieces)/.75 lb.)

**Directions:**

1. Heat the Air Fryer and wait for it to reach 285º F.
2. Shake the salt over the salmon and add them to the fryer basket with the olive oil to air-fry for 10 minutes.
3. Whisk the yogurt, salt, and dill.
4. Serve the salmon with the sauce with your favorite sides.

Cal 340 | Carb 5g | Fat 16g | Protein 32 g

# Crumbled Fish

**Preparation Time:** 5 minutes | **Cooking Time:** 15 minutes | **Serves:** 4

**Ingredients:**

- Breadcrumbs (.5 cup)
- Vegetable oil (4 tbsp.)
- Egg (1)
- Fish fillets (4)
- Lemon (1)

**Directions:**

1. Heat the Air Fryer to reach 350º F.
2. Whisk the oil and breadcrumbs until crumbly.
3. Dip the fish into the egg, then the crumb mixture.
4. Arrange the fish in the cooker and air-fry for 12 minutes. Garnish using the lemon.

Cal 320 | Carb 8g | Fat 10g | Protein 28 g

# Easy Crab Sticks

**Preparation Time:** 5 minutes | **Cooking Time:** 10 minutes | **Serves:** 4

**Ingredients:**

- Crab sticks (1 package)
- Cooking oil spray (as needed)

**Directions:**

1. Take each of the sticks out of the package and unroll it until the stick is flat. Tear the sheets into thirds.
2. Arrange them on the air fryer basket and lightly spritz using cooking spray. Set the timer for 10 minutes.
3. Note: If you shred the crab meat, you can cut the time in half, but they will also easily fall through the holes in the basket.

Cal 285 | Fat 12.8g | Carb 3.7g | Protein 38.1 g

# Deep Fried Prawns

**Preparation Time:** 15 minutes | **Cooking Time:** 20 minutes | **Serves:** 6

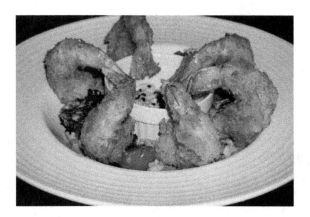

**Ingredients:**
- 12 prawns
- 2 eggs
- Flour to taste
- Breadcrumbs
- 1 tsp oil

**Direction:**
1. Remove the head of the prawns and shell carefully.
2. Pass the prawns first in the flour, then in the beaten egg and then in the breadcrumbs.
3. Preheat the air fryer for 1 minute at 300°F.
4. Add the prawns and cook for 4 minutes. If the prawns are large, cook 6 at a time.
5. Turn the prawns and cook for another 4 minutes.
6. They should be served with a yogurt or mayonnaise sauce.

Cal 2385.1 | Fat 23g | Carb 52.3g | Sugar 0.1g | Protein 21.4g

# Zucchini with Tuna

**Preparation Time:** 10 minutes | **Cooking Time:** 30 minutes | **Serves:** 4

**Ingredients:**
- 4 medium zucchinis
- 120g of tuna in oil (canned) drained
- 30g grated cheese

- 1 tsp pine nuts
- Salt, pepper to taste

**Direction**:
1. Cut the zucchini in half laterally and empty it with a small spoon (set aside the pulp that will be used for filling); place them in the basket.
2. In a food processor, put the zucchini pulp, drained tuna, pine nuts and grated cheese. Mix everything until you get a homogeneous and dense mixture.
3. Fill the zucchini. Set the air fryer to 350°F.
4. Simmer for 20 min. depending on the size of the zucchini. Let cool before serving.

Cal 389 | Carb 10g | Fat 29g | Sugars 5g | Protein 23g

## Caramelized Salmon Fillet

**Preparation Time:** 5 minutes | **Cooking Time:** 25 minutes | **Serves:** 4

**Ingredients:**
- 2 salmon fillets
- 60g cane sugar
- 4 tbsp soy sauce
- 50g sesame seeds
- Unlimited Ginger

**Direction**:
1. Preheat the air fryer at 350°F for 5 minutes.
2. Put the sugar and soy sauce in the basket.
3. Cook everything for 5 minutes.
4. In the meantime, wash the fish well, pass it through sesame to cover it completely and place it inside the tank and add the fresh ginger.
5. Cook for 12 minutes.
6. Turn the fish over and finish cooking for another 8 minutes.

Cal 569 |Fat 14.9 g| Carb 40g | Sugars 27.6g | Protein 66.9g

## Mussels with Pepper

**Preparation Time:** 15 minutes | **Cooking Time:** 20 minutes | **Serves:** 5

**Ingredients:**
- 700g mussels
- 1 clove garlic
- 1 tsp oil
- Pepper to taste
- Parsley Taste

**Direction**:

1. Clean and scrape the mold cover and remove the byssus (the "beard" that comes out of the mold).
2. Pour the oil, clean the mussels and the crushed garlic in the air fryer basket. Set the temperature to 390°F and simmer for 12 minutes. Towards the end of cooking, add black pepper and chopped parsley.
3. Finally, distribute the mussel juice well at the bottom of the basket, stirring the basket.

Cal 150 | Carb 2g | Fat 8g | Sugars 0g | Protein 15g

# Monkfish with Olives and Capers

**Preparation Time:** 25 minutes | **Cooking Time:** 40 minutes | **Serves:** 4

**Ingredients:**

- 1 monkfish
- 10 cherry tomatoes
- 50 g cailletier olives
- 5 capers

**Direction**:

1. Spread aluminum foil inside the air fryer basket and place the monkfish clean and skinless.
2. Add chopped tomatoes, olives, capers, oil, and salt.
3. Set the temperature to 320°F. Cook the monkfish for about 40 minutes.

Cal 404 | Fat 29g | Carb 36g | Sugars 7g | Protein 24g

# Shrimp, Zucchini and Cherry Tomato

**Preparation Time:** 5 minutes | **Cooking Time:** 30 minutes | **Serves:** 4

**Ingredients:**

- 2 zucchinis
- 300 shrimp
- 7 cherry tomatoes
- Salt and pepper to taste
- 1 clove garlic

**Direction**:

1. Pour the oil in the air fryer, add the garlic clove and diced zucchini.
2. Cook for 15 minutes at 300°F.

3. Add the shrimp and the pieces of tomato, salt, and spices.
4. Cook for another 5 to 10 minutes or until the shrimp water evaporates.

Cal 214.3 | Fat 8.6g | Carb 7.8g | Sugars 4.8g | Protein 27.0g

# Salted Marinated Salmon

**Preparation Time:** 10 minutes | **Cooking Time:** 30 minutes | **Serves:** 4

**Ingredients:**
- 500g salmon fillet
- 1 kg coarse salt

**Direction**:
1. Place the baking paper on the air fryer basket and the salmon on top (skin side up) covered with coarse salt. Set the air fryer to 300°F.
2. Cook everything for 25 to 30 minutes. At the end of cooking, remove the salt from the fish and serve with a drizzle of oil.

Cal 290 | Fat 13g | Carb 3g | Fiber 0g | Protein 40g

# Salmon with Pistachio Bark

**Preparation Time:** 10 minutes | **Cooking Time:** 30 minutes | **Serves:** 4

**Ingredients:**
- 600 g salmon fillet
- 50g pistachios
- Salt to taste

**Direction**:
5. Put the parchment paper on the bottom of the air fryer basket and place the salmon fillet in it (it can be cooked whole or already divided into four portions).
6. Cut the pistachios in thick pieces; grease the top of the fish, salt (little because the pistachios are already salted) and cover everything with the pistachios.
7. Set the air fryer to 350°F and simmer for 25 minutes.

Cal 371.7 | Fat 21.8g | Carb 9.4g | Sugars 2.2g | Protein 34.7g

# Sautéed Trout with Almonds

**Preparation Time:** 35 minutes | **Cooking Time:** 20 minutes | **Serves:** 4

**Ingredients:**

- 700 g salmon trout
- 15 black peppercorns
- Dill leaves to taste
- 30g almonds
- Salt to taste

**Direction:**

1. Cut the trout into cubes and marinate it for half an hour with the rest of the ingredients (except salt).
2. Cook in air fryer for 17 minutes at 320°F. Pour a drizzle of oil and serve.

Cal 238.5 | Fat 20.1g | Carb 11.5g | Sugars 1.0g | Protein4.0 g

# Air Fryer Shrimp a La Bang

**Preparation Time:** 10 minutes | **Cooking Time:** 12 minutes | **Serves:** 2

**Ingredients:**

- 1/2 cup mayonnaise
- 1/4 cup sweet chili sauce
- 1 tablespoon. sriracha sauce
- 1/4 cup all-purpose flour
- 1 cup panko bread crumbs
- Raw shrimp: 1 pound, peeled and deveined
- 1 leaf lettuce
- 2green, chopped onions or to taste (optional)

**Directions:**

1. Set temperature of air fryer to 400°F.
2. In a bowl, stir in mayonnaise, chili sauce, and sriracha sauce until smooth. Put some bang sauce, if desired, in a separate bowl for dipping.
3. Take a plate and place flour on it. Use a separate plate and place panko bread crumbs on it.
4. First coat the shrimp with flour, then mayonnaise mixture, then panko. Place shrimp covered on a baking sheet.
5. Place shrimp, without overcrowding, in the air fryer basket.
6. Cook for approximately 12 minutes. Repeat with shrimp leftover.
7. Use lettuce wraps for serving, garnished with green onion.

Cal 415 | Fat 23.9g | Carb 32.7g | Protein 23.9 g

# Breaded Cod Sticks

**Preparation Time:** 5 minutes | **Cooking Time:** 20 minutes | **Serves:** 4

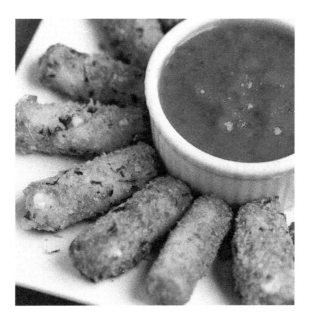

**Ingredients:**

- Large eggs (2)
- Milk (3 tbsp.)
- Breadcrumbs (2 cups)
- Almond flour (1 cup)
- Cod (1 lb.)

**Directions:**

1. Heat the Air Fryer at 350º F.
2. Prepare three bowls; one with the milk and eggs, one with the breadcrumbs (salt and pepper if desired), and another with almond flour.
3. Dip the sticks in the flour, egg mixture, and breadcrumbs.
4. Place in the basket and set the timer for 12 minutes. Toss the basket halfway through the cooking process.
5. Serve with your favorite sauce.

Cal 254 | Fat 14.2g | Carb 5.7g | Protein 39.1g

# Air Fried Crumbed Fish

**Preparation Time:** 10 minutes | **Cooking Time:** 12 minutes | **Serves:** 4

**Ingredients:**

- Bread crumbs: 1 cup
- Vegetable oil: ¼ cup
- 4 Flounder fillets
- 1 Beaten egg
- 1 Sliced Lemon

**Directions:**

1. Preheat an air fryer to 350°F.
2. In a cup add the bread crumbs and the oil. Stir until the mixture becomes crumbly and loose.
3. Dip the fish fillets in the egg mixture; shake off any excesses. Dip the fillets into a mixture of bread crumbs; until evenly and thoroughly coated.
4. Gently lay coated fillets in the preheated air fryer. Cook, about 12 minutes, with a fork, until fish flakes easily. Garnish with sliced lemon.

Cal 354 Cal | Fat 17.7g | Carb 22.5g | Protein 26.9 g

# Rabas

**Preparation Time:** 5 minutes | **Cooking Time:** 12 minutes | **Serves:** 4

**Ingredients:**

- 16 rabas
- 1 egg
- Breadcrumbs
- Salt, pepper, sweet paprika

**Direction:**

1. Put the rabas in the air fryer to boil for 2 minutes. Remove and dry well.
2. Beat the egg and season to taste. You can put salt, pepper and sweet paprika. Place in the egg.
3. Bread with breadcrumbs. Place in sticks.

Cal 356 | Fat 18g | Carb 5g | Protein 34g

# Honey Glazed Salmon

**Preparation Time:** 10 minutes | **Cooking Time:** 8 minutes | **Serves:** 2

**Ingredients:**

- 2 (6-oz.) salmon fillets
- Salt, as required
- 2 tablespoons honey

**Directions:**
1. Sprinkle the salmon fillets with salt and then, coat with honey.
2. Take to your Kalorik Maxx Air Fryer at 355°F for 8 minutes.
3. Serve hot.

Cal 289 | Fat 10.5g | Carb 17.3g | Protein 33.1 g

## Sweet & Sour Glazed Salmon

**Preparation Time:** 12 minutes | **Cooking Time:** 20 minutes | **Serves:** 2

**Ingredients:**
- 1/3 cup soy sauce
- 1/3 cup honey
- 3 teaspoons rice wine vinegar
- 1 teaspoon water
- 4 (3½-oz.) salmon fillets

**Directions:**
1. Mix the soy sauce, honey, vinegar, and water together in a bowl.
2. In another small bowl, reserve about half of the mixture.
3. Add salmon fillets in the remaining mixture and coat well.
4. Cover the bowl and refrigerate to marinate for about 2 hours.
5. Arrange the salmon fillets in greased "Air Fry Basket" and cook at 355°F for 12 minutes
6. Flip the salmon fillets once halfway through and coat with the reserved marinade after every 3 minutes. Serve hot.

Cal 462 | Fat 12.3g | Carb 49.8g | Protein 41.3 g

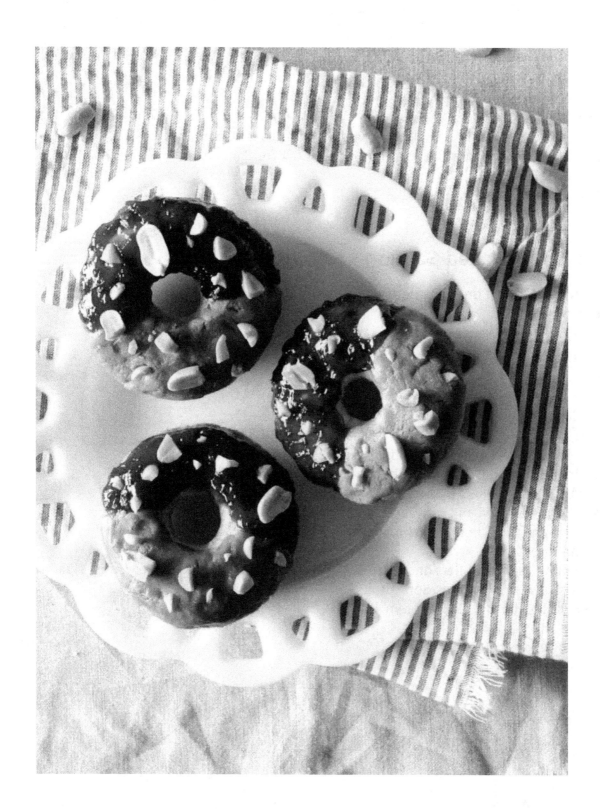

# Dessert

## Coconut Donuts

**Preparation Time:** 5 minutes | **Cooking Time:** 15 minutes | **Serves:** 4

**Ingredients:**

- 8 ounces coconut flour
- 1 egg, whisked
- and ½ tablespoons butter, melted
- 4 ounces coconut milk
- 1 teaspoon baking powder

**Directions:**

1. In a bowl, put all of the ingredients and mix well.
2. Shape donuts from this mix, place them in your air fryer's basket and cook at 370°F for 15 minutes.
3. Serve warm.

Cal 190 | Protein 6g | Fat 12g | Carb 4g

## Apple Chips

**Preparation Time:** 10 minutes | **Cooking Time:** 20 minutes | **Serves:** 2

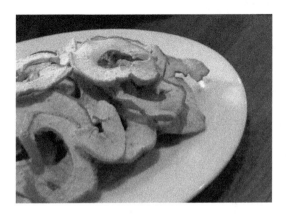

**Ingredients:**

- 1 apple, sliced thinly
- Salt to taste
- ¼ teaspoon ground cinnamon

**Directions:**

1. Preheat the air fryer to 350°F.
2. Toss the apple slices in salt and cinnamon.
3. Add to your Kalorik Maxx Air Fryer.
4. Let cool before serving.

Cal 59 | Protein 0.3g | Fat 0.2g | Carb 15.6g

## Blueberry Cream

**Preparation Time:** 4 minutes | **Cooking Time:** 20 minutes | **Serves:** 6

**Ingredients:**

- 2 cups blueberries
- Juice of ½ lemon
- 2 tablespoons water
- 1 teaspoon vanilla extract
- 2 tablespoons swerve

**Directions:**

1. In a large bowl, put all ingredients and mix well.
2. Divide this into 6 ramekins, put them in the air fryer and cook at 340°F for 20 minutes
3. Cool down and serve.

Cal 123 | Protein 3g| Fat 2g | Carb 4g

## Blackberry Chia Jam

**Preparation Time:** 10 minutes | **Cooking Time:** 30 minutes | **Serves:** 12

**Ingredients:**

- 3 cups blackberries
- ¼ cup swerve
- 4 tablespoonslemon juice
- 4 tablespoonschia seeds

**Directions:**

1. In a pan that suits the air fryer, combine all the ingredients and toss.

2. Put the pan in the fryer and cook at 300°F for 30 minutes.
3. Divide into cups and serve cold.

Cal 100 | Protein 1g | Fat 2g | Carb 3g

---

# Mixed Berries Cream

**Preparation Time:** 5 minutes | **Cooking Time:** 30 minutes | **Serves:** 6

**Ingredients:**
- 12 ounces blackberries
- 6 ounces raspberries
- 12 ounces blueberries
- ¾ cup swerve
- 2 ounces coconut cream

**Directions:**
1. In a bowl, put all the ingredients and mix well.
2. Divide this into 6 ramekins, put them in your air fryer and cook at 320°F for 30 minutes.
3. Cool down and serve it.

Cal 100 | Protein 2g | Fat 1g | Carb 2g

---

# Cinnamon-Spiced
# Acorn Squash

**Preparation Time:** 5 minutes | **Cooking Time:** 15 minutes | **Serves:** 2

**Ingredients:**
- 1 medium acorn squash, halved crosswise and deseeded
- 1 teaspoon coconut oil
- 1 teaspoon light brown sugar
- Few dashes of ground cinnamon
- Few dashes of ground nutmeg

**Directions:**
1. On a clean work surface, rub the cut sides of the acorn squash with coconut oil. Scatter with the brown sugar, cinnamon, and nutmeg.
2. Put the squash halves in the air fryer basket, cut-side up.
3. Put in the air fryer basket and cook at 325°F for 15 minutes.
4. When cooking is complete, the squash halves should be just tender when pierced in the center with a paring knife. Remove from the oven. Rest for 5 to 10 minutes and serve warm.

Cal 172 | Fat 9.8g | Carb 17.5g | Protein 3.9g

# Sweetened Plantains

**Preparation Time:** 5 minutes | **Cooking Time:** 8 minutes | **Serves:** 4

**Ingredients:**

- 2 ripe plantains, sliced
- 2 teaspoons avocado oil
- Salt to taste
- Maple syrup

**Directions:**

1. Toss the plantains in oil.
2. Season with salt.
3. Cook in the air fryer basket at 400°F for 10 minutes, shaking after 5 minutes.
4. Drizzle with maple syrup before serving.

Cal 125 | Protein 1.2g | Fat 0.6g | Carb 32g

# Pear Crisp

**Preparation Time:** 10 minutes | **Cooking Time:** 25 minutes | **Serves:** 2

**Ingredients:**

- 1 cup flour
- 1 stick vegan butter
- 1 tablespoon cinnamon
- ½ cup sugar
- 2 pears, cubed

**Directions:**

1. Mix flour and butter to form crumbly texture.
2. Add cinnamon and sugar.
3. Put the pears in the air fryer.
4. Pour and spread the mixture on top of the pears.
5. Cook at 350°F for 25 minutes.

Cal 544 | Protein 7.4g | Fat 0.9g | Carb 132.3g

# Cinnamon Rolls

**Preparation Time:** 2 hours| **Cooking Time:** 15 minutes | **Serves:** 8

**Ingredients:**

- 1 pound vegan bread dough
- ¾ cup coconut sugar

- 1 and ½ tablespoons cinnamon powder
- 2 tablespoons vegetable oil

**Directions:**
1. Roll dough on a floured working surface, shape a rectangle and brush with the oil.
2. In a bowl, mix cinnamon with sugar, stir, sprinkle this over dough, roll into a log, seal well and cut into 8 pieces.
3. Leave rolls to rise for 2 hours, place them in your air fryer's basket, cook at 350°F for 5 minutes, flip them, cook for 4 minutes more and transfer to a platter.
4. Enjoy!

Cal 170 | Protein 6g | Fat 1g | Carb 7g

## Easy Pears Dessert

**Preparation Time:** 10 minutes | **Cooking Time:** 25 minutes | **Serves:** 12

**Ingredients:**
- 6 big pears, cored and chopped
- ½ cup raisins
- 1 teaspoon ginger powder
- ¼ cup coconut sugar
- 1 teaspoon lemon zest, grated

**Directions:**
1. In a container that fits your air fryer, mix pears with raisins, ginger, sugar and lemon zest, stir, introduce in the fryer and cook at 350°F for 25 minutes.
2. Divide into bowls and serve cold.

Cal 200 | Protein 6g | Fat 3g | Carb 6g

## Raisins Cinnamon Peaches

**Preparation Time:** 10 minutes / **Cooking Time:** 15 minutes / **Serves:** 4

**Ingredients:**
- 4 peaches, cored and cut into chunks
- 1 tsp vanilla
- 1 tsp cinnamon
- ½ cup raisins
- 1 cup of water

**Directions:**
1. Put all of the ingredients in the pot and stir well.
2. Seal pot and cook on high for 15 minutes.

3. As soon as the cooking is done, let it release pressure naturally for 10 minutes then release remaining using quick release. Remove lid.
4. Stir and serve.

Cal 118 | Protein 2g | Fat 0.5g | Carb 29 g

## Sweet Bananas and Sauce

**Preparation Time:** 10 minutes | **Cooking Time:** 20 minutes | **Serves:** 4

**Ingredients:**
- Juice of ½ lemon
- 3 tablespoons agave nectar
- 1 tablespoon coconut oil
- 4 bananas, peeled and sliced diagonally
- ½ teaspoon cardamom seeds

**Directions:**
1. Arrange bananas in a pan that fits your air fryer, add agave nectar, lemon juice, oil and cardamom, introduce in the fryer and cook at 360°F for 20 minutes
2. Divide bananas and sauce between plates and serve.
3. Enjoy!

Cal 210 | Protein 3g | Fat 1g | Carb 8g

## Vanilla Strawberry Mix

**Preparation Time:** 10 minutes | **Cooking Time:** 20 minutes | **Serves:** 10

**Ingredients:**
- 2 tablespoons lemon juice
- 2 pounds strawberries
- 4 cups coconut sugar
- 1 teaspoon cinnamon powder
- 1 teaspoon vanilla extract

**Directions:**
1. In a pot that fits your air fryer, mix strawberries with coconut sugar, lemon juice, cinnamon and vanilla, stir gently, introduce in the fryer and cook at 350°F for 20 minutes
2. Divide into bowls and serve cold.

Cal 140 | Protein 2g | Fat 0g | Carb 5g

# Cinnamon Apples and Mandarin Sauce

**Preparation Time:** 10 minutes | **Cooking Time:** 20 minutes | **Serves:** 4

**Ingredients:**

- 4 apples, cored, peeled and cored
- 2 cups mandarin juice
- ¼ cup maple syrup
- 2 teaspoons cinnamon powder
- 1 tablespoon ginger, grated

**Directions:**

1. In a pot that fits your air fryer, mix apples with mandarin juice, maple syrup, cinnamon and ginger, introduce in the fryer and cook at 365°F for 20 minutes
2. Divide apples mix between plates and serve warm.
3. Enjoy!

Cal 170 | Protein 4g | Fat 1g | Carb 6g

# Chocolate Vanilla Bars

**Preparation Time:** 10 minutes | **Cooking Time:** 7 minutes | **Serves:** 12

**Ingredients:**

- 1 cup sugar free and vegan chocolate chips
- 2 tablespoons coconut butter
- 2/3 cup coconut cream
- tablespoons stevia
- ¼ teaspoon vanilla extract

**Directions:**

1. Put the cream in a bowl, add stevia, butter and chocolate chips and stir
2. Leave aside for 5 minutes, stir well and mix the vanilla.
3. Transfer the mix into a lined baking sheet, introduce in your air fryer and cook at 356°F for 7 minutes.
4. Leave the mix aside to cool down, slice and serve.
5. Enjoy!

Cal 120 | Protein 1g | Fat 5g | Carb 6g

# Raspberry Bars

**Preparation Time:** 10 minutes | **Cooking Time:** 6 minutes | **Serves:** 12

**Ingredients:**
- ½ cup coconut butter, melted
- ½ cup coconut oil
- ½ cup raspberries, dried
- ¼ cup swerve
- ½ cup coconut, shredded

**Directions:**
1. In your food processor, blend dried berries very well.
2. In a bowl that fits your air fryer, mix oil with butter, swerve, coconut and raspberries, toss well, introduce in the fryer and cook at 320°F for 6 minutes.
3. Spread this on a lined baking sheet, keep in the fridge for an hour, slice and serve.
4. Enjoy!

Cal 164 | Protein 2g | Fat 22g | Carb 4g

## Cocoa Berries Cream

**Preparation Time:** 10 minutes | **Cooking Time:** 10 minutes | **Serves:** 4

**Ingredients:**
- 3 tablespoons cocoa powder
- 14 ounces coconut cream
- 1 cup blackberries
- 1 cup raspberries
- 2 tablespoons stevia

**Directions:**
1. In a bowl, whisk cocoa powder with stevia and cream and stir.
2. Add raspberries and blackberries, toss gently, transfer to a pan that fits your air fryer, introduce in the fryer and cook at 350°F for 10 minutes.
3. Divide into bowls and serve cold.
4. Enjoy!

Cal 205 | Protein 2g | Fat 34g | Carb 6g

## Cocoa Pudding

**Preparation Time:** 10 minutes | **Cooking Time:** 20 minutes | **Serves:** 2

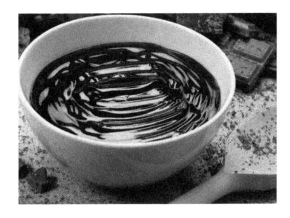

**Ingredients:**
- 2 tablespoons water
- ½ tablespoon agar
- 4 tablespoons stevia
- 4 tablespoons cocoa powder
- 2 cups coconut milk, hot

**Directions:**
1. In a bowl, mix milk with stevia and cocoa powder and stir well.
2. In a bowl, mix agar with water, stir well, add to the cocoa mix, stir and transfer to a pudding pan that fits your air fryer.
3. Introduce in the fryer and cook at 356°F for 20 minutes.
4. Serve the pudding cold.
5. Enjoy!

Cal 170 | Protein 3g | Fat 2g | Carb 4g

# Blueberry Coconut Crackers

**Preparation Time:** 10 minutes | **Cooking Time:** 30 minutes | **Serves:** 12

**Ingredients:**
- ½ cup coconut butter
- ½ cup coconut oil, melted
- 1 cup blueberries
- 3 tablespoons coconut sugar

**Directions:**
1. In a pot that fits your air fryer, mix coconut butter with coconut oil, raspberries and sugar, toss, introduce in the fryer and cook at 367°F for 30 minutes
2. Spread on a lined baking sheet, keep in the fridge for a few hours, slice crackers and serve.

3. Enjoy!

Cal 174 | Protein 7g | Fat 5g | Carb 4g

## Cauliflower Pudding

**Preparation Time:** 10 minutes | **Cooking Time:** 30 minutes | *Serves:* 4

**Ingredients:**
- 2½ cups water
- 1 cup coconut sugar
- 2 cups cauliflower rice
- 2 cinnamon sticks
- ½ cup coconut, shredded

**Directions:**
1. In a pot that fits your air fryer, mix water with coconut sugar, cauliflower rice, cinnamon and coconut, stir, introduce in the fryer and cook at 365°F for 30 minutes
2. Divide pudding into cups and serve cold.
3. Enjoy!

Cal 203 | Protein 4g | Fat 4g | Carb 9g

## Sweet Vanilla Rhubarb

**Preparation Time:** 10 minutes | **Cooking Time:** 10 minutes | **Serves:** 4

**Ingredients:**
- 5 cups rhubarb, chopped
- 2 tablespoons coconut butter, melted
- 1/3 cup water
- 1 tablespoon stevia
- 1 teaspoon vanilla extract

**Directions:**
1. Put rhubarb, ghee, water, stevia and vanilla extract in a pan that fits your air fryer, introduce in the fryer and cook at 365°F for 10 minutes
2. Divide into small bowls and serve cold.
3. Enjoy!

Cal 103 | Protein 2g | Fat 2g | Carb 6g

# Blueberry Jam

**Preparation Time:** 10 minutes | **Cooking Time:** 11 minutes | **Serves:** 2

**Ingredients:**
- ½ pound blueberries
- 1/3 pound sugar
- Zest from ½ lemon, grated
- ½ tablespoon butter
- A pinch of cinnamon powder

**Directions:**
1. Put the blueberries in your blender, pulse them well, strain, transfer to your pressure cooker, add sugar, lemon zest and cinnamon, stir, cover and simmer on sauté mode for 3 minutes.
2. Add butter, stir, cover the fryer and cook on High for 8 minutes.
3. Transfer to a jar and serve.

Cal 211 | Protein 5g | Fat 3g | Carb 6g

# Pineapple Pudding

**Preparation Time:** 10 minutes | **Cooking Time:** 5 minutes | **Serves:** 8

**Ingredients:**
- 1 tablespoon avocado oil
- 1 cup rice
- 14 ounces milk
- Sugar to the taste
- 8 ounces canned pineapple, chopped

**Directions:**
1. In your air fryer, mix oil, milk and rice, stir, cover and cook on High for 3 minutes.
2. Add sugar and pineapple, stir, cover and cook on High for 2 minutes more.
3. Divide into dessert bowls and serve.

Cal 154 | Protein 8g | Fat 4g | Carb 14g

# Plum Jam

**Preparation Time:** 20 minutes | **Cooking Time:** 8 minutes | **Serves:** 12

**Ingredients:**
- 3 pounds plums, stones removed and roughly chopped
- 2 tablespoons lemon juice
- 2 pounds sugar

- 1 teaspoon vanilla extract
- 3 ounces water

**Directions:**
1. In your air fryer, mix plums with sugar and vanilla extract, stir and leave aside for 20 minutes
2. Add lemon juice and water, stir, cover and cook on High for 8 minutes.
3. Divide into bowls and serve cold.

Cal 191 | Protein 13g | Fat 3g | Carb 12g

# Coconut Pancake

**Preparation Time:** 10 minutes | **Cooking Time:** 20 minutes | **Serves:** 4

**Ingredients:**
- 2 cups self-rising flour
- 2 tablespoons sugar
- 2 eggs
- 1 and ½ cups coconut milk
- A drizzle of olive oil

**Directions:**
1. In a bowl, mix eggs with sugar, milk and flour and whisk until you obtain a batter.
2. Grease your air fryer with the oil, add the batter, spread into the pot, cover and cook on Low for 20 minutes.
3. Slice pancake, divide between plates and serve cold.

Cal 162 | Protein 8g | Fat 3g | Carb 7g

# Apples and Red Grape Juice

**Preparation Time:** 10 minutes | **Cooking Time;** 10 minutes | **Serves:** 2

**Ingredients:**
- 2 apples
- ½ cup natural red grape juice
- 2 tablespoons raisins
- 1 teaspoon cinnamon powder
- ½ tablespoons sugar

**Directions:**
1. Put the apples in your air fryer, add grape juice, raisins, cinnamon and stevia, toss a bit, cover and cook on High for 10 minutes.

2. Divide into 2 bowls and serve.

Cal 110 | Protein 3g | Fat 1g | Carb 3g

# Cherries and Rhubarb Bowls

**Preparation Time:** 10 minutes / **Cooking Time:** 35 minutes /**Servings:** 4

**Ingredients:**
- 2 cups cherries, pitted and halved
- 1 cup rhubarb, sliced
- 1 cup apple juice
- 2tablespoons sugar
- ½ cup raisins.

**Directions:**
1. In a pot that fits your air fryer, combine the cherries with the rhubarb and the other ingredients, toss, cook at 330°F for 35 minutes, divide into bowls, cool down and serve.

Cal 212 | Protein 7g | Fat 8g | Carbs 13g

# Coconut and Avocado Pudding

**Preparation Time:** 2 hours| **Cooking Time:** 2 minutes | **Serves:** 3

**Ingredients:**
- ½ cup avocado oil
- 4 tablespoons sugar
- 1 tablespoon cocoa powder
- 14 ounces canned coconut milk
- 1 avocado, pitted, peeled and chopped

**Directions:**
1. In a bowl, mix oil with cocoa powder and half of the sugar, stir well, transfer to a lined container, keep in the fridge for 1 hour and chop into small pieces.
2. In your air fryer, mix coconut milk with avocado and the rest of the sugar, blend using an immersion blender, cover cooker and cook on High for 2 minutes.
3. Add chocolate chips, stir, divide pudding into bowls and keep in the fridge until you serve it.

Cal 140 | Protein 4g | Fat 3g | Carb 3g

# SUPER FAST 5-Minutes Recipes

## Lemony Apple Bites

**Preparation Time:** 5 minutes | **Cooking Time:** 5 minutes | **Serves:** 4

**Ingredients:**

- big apples, cored, peeled and cubed
- teaspoons lemon juice
- ½ cup caramel sauce

**Directions:**

1. In your air fryer, mix all the ingredients; toss well.
2. Cook at 340°F for 5 minutes.
3. Divide into cups and serve as a snack.

Cal 180 | Fat 4g | Fiber 3g | Carb 10g | Protein 3g

## Asparagus with Almonds

**Preparation Time:** 5 minutes | **Cooking Time:** 5 minutes | **Serves:** 2

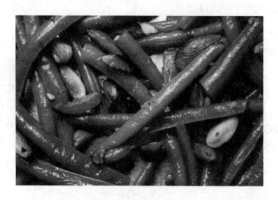

**Ingredients:**

- 9 ounces asparagus
- 1 teaspoon almond flour
- 1 tablespoon almond flakes
- ¼ teaspoon salt
- 1 teaspoon olive oil

**Directions:**

1. Combine the almond flour and almond flakes; stir the mixture well.
2. Sprinkle the asparagus with the olive oil and salt.
3. Shake it gently and coat in the almond flour mixture.
4. Place the asparagus in the air fryer basket and cook at 400°F for 5 minutes, stirring halfway through.
5. Then cool a little and serve.

Cal 143 | Fat 11g | Fiber 4.6g | Carb 8.6g | Protein 6.4g

## Sky-High Roasted Corn

**Preparation Time:** 5 minutes | **Cooking Time:** 5 minutes | **Serves:** 4

**Ingredients:**

- 4 ears of husk-less corn
- 1 tablespoon of olive oil
- 1 teaspoon of salt
- 1 teaspoon of black pepper

**Directions:**

1. Heat up your air fryer to 400°F.
2. Sprinkle the ears of corn with the olive oil, salt and black pepper.
3. Place it inside your air fryer and cook it for 5 minutes at 400°F.
4. Serve and enjoy!

Cal 100 | Fat 1g | Protein 3g | Fiber 3g | Carb 22g

## Pleasant Air-Fried Eggplant

**Preparation Time:** 5 minutes | **Cooking Time:** 5 minutes | **Serves:** 4

**Ingredients:**

- 2 thinly sliced or chopped into chunks eggplants
- 1 teaspoon of salt
- 1 teaspoon of black pepper
- 1 cup of rice flour
- 1 cup of white wine

**Directions:**

1. Using a bowl, add the rice flour, white wine and mix properly until it gets smooth.
2. Add the salt, black pepper and stir again.
3. Dredge the eggplant slices or chunks into the batter and remove any excess batter.
4. Heat up your air fryer to 390°F.
5. Grease your air fryer basket with a nonstick cooking spray.
6. Add the eggplant slices or chunks into your air fryer and cook it for 5 minutes or until it has a golden brown and crispy texture, while still shaking it occasionally.
7. Carefully remove it from your air fryer and allow it to cool off. Serve and enjoy!

Cal 380 | Fat 15g | Protein 13g | Fiber 6.1g | Carb 51g

# Garlic Prawn

**Preparation Time:** 5 minutes | **Cooking Time:** 5 minutes | **Serves:** 4

**Ingredients:**
- 15 fresh prawns
- 1 tablespoon olive oil
- 1 teaspoon chili powder
- 1 tablespoon black pepper
- 1 tablespoon chili sauce
- 1 garlic clove, minced
- Salt as needed

**Directions:**
1. Preheat your Air Fryer to 356°F
2. Wash prawns thoroughly and rinse them
3. Take a mixing bowl and add washed prawn, chili powder, oil, garlic, pepper, chili sauce and stir the mix
4. Transfer prawn to Air Fryer and cook for 5 minutes
5. Serve and enjoy!

Cal 140 | Fat 10g | Carb 5g | Protein 8g

# Zucchini Cubes

**Preparation Time:** 5 minutes | **Cooking Time:** 5 minutes | **Serves:** 2

**Ingredients:**
- 1 zucchini
- ½ teaspoon ground black pepper
- 1 teaspoon oregano
- 2 tablespoons chicken stock

- ½ teaspoon coconut oil

**Directions:**
1. Chop the zucchini into cubes.
2. Combine the ground black pepper, and oregano; stir the mixture.
3. Sprinkle the zucchini cubes with the spice mixture and stir well.
4. After this, sprinkle the vegetables with the chicken stock.
5. Place the coconut oil in the air fryer basket and preheat it to 360°F for 20 seconds.
6. Then add the zucchini cubes and cook the vegetables for 5 minutes at 390°F, stirring halfway through.
7. Transfer to serving plates and enjoy!

Cal 30 | Fat 1.5g | Fiber 1.6g | Carb 4.3g | Protein 1.4g

# Turmeric Cauliflower Rice

**Preparation Time:** 5 minutes | **Cooking Time:** 5 minutes | **Serves:** 6

**Ingredients:**
- oz chive stems
- tablespoon butter
- 1 teaspoon salt
- 1-pound cauliflower
- 1 teaspoon turmeric
- 1 teaspoon minced garlic
- 1 teaspoon ground ginger
- 1 cup chicken stock

**Directions:**
1. Wash the cauliflower and chop it roughly.
2. Then place the chopped cauliflower in the blender and blend it till you get the rice texture of the cauliflower.
3. Transfer the cauliflower rice to the mixing bowl and add the diced chives.
4. After this, sprinkle the vegetable mixture with the salt, turmeric, minced garlic, and ground ginger. Mix it up.
5. Preheat the air fryer to 370°F.
6. Put the cauliflower rice mixture there. Add the butter and chicken stock.
7. Cook the cauliflower rice for 5 minutes.
8. When the time is over – remove the cauliflower rice from the air fryer and strain the excess liquid.
9. Stir it gently. Enjoy!

Cal 82 | Fat 1g | Fiber 0g | Carb 1.4g | Protein 0g

# Roasted Garlic Head

**Preparation Time:** 5 minutes | **Cooking Time:** 5 minutes | **Serves:** 4

**Ingredients:**

- 1-pound garlic head
- 1 tablespoon olive oil
- 1 teaspoon thyme

**Directions:**

1. Cut the ends of the garlic head and place it in the air fryer basket.
2. Then sprinkle the garlic head with the olive oil and thyme.
3. Cook the garlic head for 5 minutes at 400°F.
4. When the garlic head is cooked, it should be soft and aromatic.
5. Serve immediately.

Cal 200 | Fat 4.1g | Fiber 2.5g | Carb 37.7g | Protein 7.2g

# Pepperoni Chips

**Preparation Time: 2 minutes | Cooking Time: 5 minutes | Serves: 6**

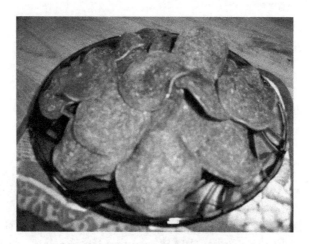

**Ingredients :**

- oz pepperoni slices

**Directions :**

1 Place one batch of pepperoni slices in the air fryer oven basket.

2 Cook for 5 minutes at 360°F.

3 Cook remaining pepperoni slices using same steps.

4 Serve and enjoy.

Cal 51 | Fat 1g | Carb 2g | Sugar 1.3g | Protein 0g

# Shirataki Noodles

**Preparation Time:** 5 minutes | **Cooking Time:** 5 minutes | **Serves:** 4

**Ingredients:**

- cups water
- 1 teaspoon salt
- 1 tablespoon Italian seasoning
- 8 ozshirataki noodles

**Directions:**

1 Preheat the air fryer to 365°F.

2 Pour the water in the air fryer basket tray and preheat it for 3 minutes.

3 Then add the shirataki noodles, salt, and Italian seasoning.

4 Cook the shirataki noodles for 1 minute at the same temperature.

5 Then strain the noodles and cook them for 2 minutes more at 360°F.

6 When the shirataki noodles are cooked – let them chill for 1-2 minutes.

7 Stir the noodles gently.

8 Serve it!

Cal 16 | Fat 1g| Fiber 0g | Carb 1.4g | Protein 0g

# Yams with Dill

**Preparation Time:** 5 minutes | **Cooking Time:** 5 minutes | **Serves:** 2

**Ingredients:**

- 2 yams
- 1 tablespoon fresh dill
- 1 teaspoon coconut oil
- ½ teaspoon minced garlic

**Directions:**

1. Wash the yams carefully and cut them into halves.
2. Sprinkle the yam halves with the coconut oil and then rub with the minced garlic.
3. Place the yams in the air fryer basket and cook for 5 minutes at 400°F.
4. After this, mash the yams gently with a fork and then sprinkle with the fresh dill.
5. Serve the yams immediately.

Cal 25 | Fat 2.3g | Fiber 0.2g | Carb 1.2g | Protein 0.4g

# Honey Onions

**Preparation Time:** 5 minutes | **Cooking Time:** 5 minutes | **Serves:** 2

**Ingredients:**

- 2 large white onions
- 1 tablespoon raw honey
- 1 teaspoon water
- 1 tablespoon paprika

**Directions:**

1. Peel the onions and using a knife, make cuts in the shape of a cross.
2. Then combine the raw honey and water; stir.
3. Add the paprika and stir the mixture until smooth.
4. Place the onions in the air fryer basket and sprinkle them with the honey mixture.
5. Cook the onions for 5 minutes at 380°F.
6. When the onions are cooked, they should be soft.
7. Transfer the cooked onions to serving plates and serve.

Cal 102 | Fat 0.6g | Fiber 4.5g | Carb 24.6g | Protein 2.2g

# Delightful Roasted Garlic Slices

**Preparation Time:** 5 minutes | **Cooking Time:** 5 minutes | **Serves:** 4

**Ingredients:**

- 1 teaspoon coconut oil
- ½ teaspoon dried cilantro
- ¼ teaspoon cayenne pepper
- 12 ounces garlic cloves, peeled

**Directions:**

1. Sprinkle the garlic cloves with the cayenne pepper and dried cilantro.
2. Mix the garlic up with the spices, and then transfer to your Kalorik Maxx Air Fryer basket.
3. Add the coconut oil and cook the garlic for 5 minutes at 400°F, stirring halfway through.
4. When the garlic cloves are done, transfer them to serving plates and serve.

Cal 137 | Fat 1.6g | Fiber 1.8g | Carb 28.2g | Protein 5.4g

# Apple Hand Pies

**Preparation Time:** 5 Minutes | **Cooking Time:** 5 Minutes | **Serves:** 6

**Ingredients:**

- 15-ounces no-sugar-added apple pie filling
- 1 store-bought crust

**Directions:**

1 Lay out pie crust and slice into equal-sized squares.

2 Place 2 tablespoon filling into each square and seal crust with a fork.

3 Pour into the Oven rack/basket. Place the Rack on the middle-shelf of the Air Fryer Oven. Set temperature to 390°F, and set time to 5 minutes until golden in color.

Cal 278 | Fat 10g | Protein 5g| Sugar 4g

## Roasted Mushrooms

**Preparation Time:**5 minutes | **Cooking Time:** 5 minutes | **Serves:** 2

**Ingredients:**
- 12 ounces mushroom hats
- ¼ cup fresh dill, chopped
- ¼ teaspoon onion, chopped
- 1 teaspoon olive oil
- ¼ teaspoon turmeric

**Directions:**
1. Combine the chopped dill and onion.
2. Add the turmeric and stir the mixture.
3. After this, add the olive oil and mix until homogenous.
4. Then fill the mushroom hats with the dill mixture and place them in the air fryer basket.
5. Cook the mushrooms for 5 minutes at 400°F.
6. When the vegetables are cooked, let them cool to room temperature before serving.

Cal 73 | Fat 3.1g | Fiber 2.6g | Carb 9.2g | Protein 6.6g

## Mashed Yams

**Preparation Time:** 5 minutes | **Cooking Time:** 5 minutes | **Serves:** 5

**Ingredients:**
- 1 pound yams
- 1 teaspoon olive oil
- 1 tablespoon almond milk
- ¾ teaspoon salt
- 1 teaspoon dried parsley

**Directions:**
1. Peel the yams and chop.

2.  Place the chopped yams in the air fryer basket and sprinkle with the salt and dried parsley.
3.  Add the olive oil and stir the mixture.
4.  Cook the yams at 400°F for 5 minutes, stirring twice during cooking.
5.  When the yams are done, blend them well with a hand blender until smooth.
6.  Add the almond milk and stir carefully.
7.  Serve, and enjoy!

Cal 120 | Fat 1.8g | Fiber 3.6g | Carb 25.1g | Protein 1.4g

## Beef and Mango Skewers

**Preparation Time:** 5 minutes | **Cooking Time:** 5 minutes | **Serves:** 4

**Ingredients:**

- ¾ pound beef sirloin tip, cut into 1-inch cubes
- 2 tablespoons balsamic vinegar
- 1 tablespoon olive oil
- 1 tablespoon honey
- ½ teaspoon dried marjoram
- Pinch salt
- Freshly ground black pepper
- 1 mango

**Directions:**

1.  Put the beef cubes in a medium bowl and add the balsamic vinegar, olive oil, honey, marjoram, salt, and pepper. Mix well, and then massage the marinade into the beef with your hands. Set aside.
2.  To prepare the mango, stand it on end and cut the skin off, using a sharp knife. Then carefully cut around the oval pit to remove the flesh. Cut the mango into 1-inch cubes.
3.  Thread metal skewers alternating with three beef cubes and two mango cubes.
4.  Grill the skewers in the air fryer basket for 5 minutes or until the beef is browned and at least 145°F.

Cal 242 | Fat 9g | Carb 13g | Protein 26g

## Cheese Bacon Jalapeno Poppers

**Preparation Time:** 5 minutes | **Cooking Time:** 5 minutes | **Serves:** 5

**Ingredients:**

- fresh jalapeno peppers, cut in half and remove seeds
- bacon slices, cooked and crumbled
- 1/4 cup cheddar cheese, shredded

6 oz cream cheese, softened**Directions:**

1 In a bowl, combine together bacon, cream cheese, and cheddar cheese.
2 Stuff each jalapeno half with bacon cheese mixture.
3 Spray air fryer oven basket with cooking spray.
4 Place stuffed jalapeno halved in air fryer oven basket and cook at 370°F for 5 minutes.
5 Serve and enjoy.

Cal 195 | Fat 17.3g | Carb 3.2g | Sugar 1g | Protein 7.2 g

## Fried Leeks

**Preparation Time:** 5 minutes | **Cooking Time:** 5 minutes | **Serves:** 4

**Ingredients:**
- 4 leeks; ends cut off and halved
- 1 tbsp. butter; melted
- 1 tbsp. lemon juice
- Salt and black pepper to the taste

**Directions:**
1. Coat leeks with melted butter, flavor with salt and pepper, put in your air fryer and cook at 350°F, for 5 minutes.
2. Arrange on a platter, drizzle lemon juice all over and serve

Cal 100 | Fat 4g | Fiber 2g | Carb 6g | Protein 2g

## Crunchy Bacon Bites

**Preparation Time:** 5 minutes | **Cooking Time:** 5 minutes | **Serves:** 4

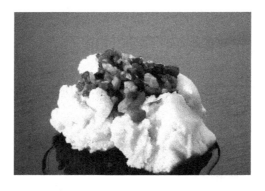

**Ingredients:**

- bacon strips, cut into small pieces
- 1/2 cup pork rinds, crushed
- 1/4 cup hot sauce

**Directions:**

1 Add bacon pieces in a bowl.

2 Add hot sauce and toss well.

3 Add crushed pork rinds and toss until bacon pieces are well coated.

4 Transfer bacon pieces in air fryer oven basket and cook at 350°F for 5minutes.

5 Serve and enjoy.

Cal 112 | Fat 9.7g | Carb 0.3g | Sugar 0.2g | Protein 5.2g

## Brussels Sprouts and Tomatoes Mix

**Preparation Time:** 5 minutes | **Cooking Time:** 5 minutes | **Serves:** 4

**Ingredients:**

- 1 lb. Brussels sprouts; trimmed
- 6 cherry tomatoes; halved
- 1/4 cup green onions; chopped.
- 1 tbsp. olive oil
- Salt and black pepper to the taste

**Directions:**

1. Season Brussels sprouts with salt and pepper, put them in your air fryer and cook at 350°F, for 5 minutes
2. Transfer them to a bowl, add salt, pepper, cherry tomatoes, green onions and olive oil, toss well and serve.

Cal 121 | Fat 4g | Fiber 4g | Carb 11g | Protein 4g

## Radish Hash Recipe

**Preparation Time:** 5 minutes | **Cooking Time:** 5 minutes | **Serves:** 4

**Ingredients:**

- 1/2 tsp. onion powder
- 1/3 cup parmesan; grated
- 4 eggs
- 1 lb. radishes; sliced

- Salt and black pepper to the taste

**Directions:**
1. In a bowl mix radishes with salt, pepper, onion, eggs and parmesan and stir well
2. Transfer radishes to a pan that fits your air fryer and cook at 350°F, for 5 minutes
3. Divide hash on plates and serve.

Cal 80 | Fat 5g | Fiber 2g | Carb 5g | Protein 7g

# Broccoli Salad Recipe

**Preparation Time:** 5 minutes | **Cooking Time:** 5 minutes | **Serves:** 4

**Ingredients:**
- 1 broccoli head; florets separated
- 1 tbsp. Chinese rice wine vinegar
- 1 tbsp. peanut oil
- 6 garlic cloves; minced
- Salt and black pepper to the taste

**Directions:**
1. In a bowl mix broccoli with salt, pepper and half of the oil, toss, transfer to your air fryer and cook at 350°F, for 5 minutes; shaking the fryer halfway
2. Transfer broccoli to a salad bowl, add the rest of the peanut oil, garlic and rice vinegar, toss really well and serve.

Cal 121 | Fat 3g | Fiber 4g | Carb 4g | Protein 4g

# Parmesan Broccoli and Asparagus

**Preparation Time:** 5 minutes | **Cooking Time:** 5 minutes | **Serves:** 4

**Ingredients:**
- 1 broccoli head, florets separated
- ½ pound asparagus, trimmed
- Juice of 1 lime
- Salt and black pepper to the taste
- 2 tablespoons olive oil
- 3 tablespoons parmesan, grated

**Directions:**
1. In a small bowl, combine the asparagus with the broccoli and all the other ingredients except the parmesan, toss, transfer to your air fryer's basket and cook at 400°F for 5 minutes.
2. Divide between plates, sprinkle the parmesan on top and serve.

Cal 172 | Fat 5g | Fiber 2g | Carb 4g | Protein 9g

## Butter Broccoli Mix

**Preparation Time:** 5 minutes | **Cooking Time:** 5 minutes | **Serves:** 4

**Ingredients:**

- 1-pound broccoli florets
- A pinch of salt and black pepper
- 1 teaspoon sweet paprika
- ½ tablespoon butter, melted

**Directions:**

1. In a small bowl, combine the broccoli with the rest of the ingredients, and toss.
2. Put the broccoli in your air fryer's basket, cook at 350°F for 5 minutes, divide between plates and serve.

Cal 130 | Fat 3g | Fiber 3g | Carb 4g | Protein 8g

## Kale and Olives

**Preparation Time:** 5 minutes | **Cooking Time:** 5 minutes | **Serves:** 4

**Ingredients:**

- 1 an ½ pounds kale, torn
- 2 tablespoons olive oil
- Salt and black pepper to the taste
- 1 tablespoon hot paprika
- 2 tablespoons black olives, pitted and sliced

**Directions:**

1. In a pan that fits the air fryer, combine all the ingredients and toss.
2. Put the pan in your air fryer, cook at 370°F for 5 minutes, divide between plates and serve.

Cal 154 | Fat 3g | Fiber 2g | Carb 4g | Protein 6g

## Kale and Mushrooms Mix

**Preparation Time:** 5 minutes | **Cooking Time:** 5 minutes | **Serves:** 4

**Ingredients:**

- 1 pound brown mushrooms, sliced
- 1-pound kale, torn

- Salt and black pepper to the taste
- 2 tablespoons olive oil
- 14 ounces coconut milk

**Directions:**
1. In a pot that fits your air fryer, mix the kale with the rest of the ingredients and toss.
2. Put the pan in the fryer, cook at 380°F for 5 minutes, divide between plates and serve.

Cal 162 | Fat 4g | Fiber 1g | Carb 3g | Protein 5g

---

# Oregano Kale

**Preparation Time:** 5 minutes | **Cooking Time:** 5 minutes | **Serves:** 4

**Ingredients:**
- 1-pound kale, torn
- 1 tablespoon olive oil
- A pinch of salt and black pepper
- 2 tablespoons oregano, chopped

**Directions:**
1. In a pan that fits the air fryer, combine all the ingredients and toss.
2. Put the pan in the air fryer and cook at 380°F for 5 minutes.
3. Divide between plates and serve.

Cal 140 | Fat 3g| Fiber 2g | Carb 3g | Protein 5g

---

# Kale and Brussels Sprouts

**Preparation Time:** 5 minutes | **Cooking Time:** 5 minutes | **Serves:** 8

**Ingredients:**
- 1-pound Brussels sprouts, trimmed
- 2 cups kale, torn
- 1 tablespoon olive oil
- Salt and black pepper to the taste
- 3 ounces mozzarella, shredded

**Directions:**
1. In a pan that fits the air fryer, combine all the ingredients except the mozzarella and toss.
2. Put the pan in the air fryer and cook at 380°F for 5 minutes.
3. Divide between plates, sprinkle the cheese on top and serve.

Cal 170 | Fat 5g | Fiber 3g | Carb 4g | Protein 7g

# Spicy Kale Chips with Yogurt Sauce

**Preparation Time:** 5 minutes | **Cooking Time**: 5 minutes | **Serves:** 4

**Ingredients:**
- 1 cup Greek yogurt
- 3 tablespoons lemon juice
- 2 tablespoons honey mustard
- ½ teaspoon dried oregano
- 1 bunch curly kale
- 2 tablespoons olive oil
- ½ teaspoon salt
- ⅛ Teaspoon pepper

**Directions:**
1. In a small bowl, combine the yogurt, lemon juice, honey mustard, and oregano, and set aside.
2. Remove the stems and ribs from the kale with a sharp knife. Cut the leaves into 2- to 3-inch pieces.
3. Toss the kale with olive oil, salt, and pepper. Massage the oil into the leaves with your hands.
4. Air-fry the kale in batches until crisp, about 5 minutes, shaking the basket once during cooking time. Serve with the yogurt sauce.

Cal 154 | Fat 8g | Carb 13g | Protein 8g

# Spicy Olives and Avocado Mix

**Preparation Time:** 5 minutes | **Cooking Time**: 5 minutes | **Serves:** 4

**Ingredients:**
- 2 cups kalamata olives, pitted
- 2 small avocados, pitted, peeled and sliced
- ¼ cup cherry tomatoes, halved
- Juice of 1 lime
- 1 tablespoon coconut oil, melted

**Directions:**
1. In a pan that fits the air fryer, combine the olives with the other ingredients, toss, put the pan in your air fryer and cook at 370°F for 5 minutes.
2. Divide the mix between plates and serve.

Cal 153 | Fat 3g | Fiber 3g | Carb 4g | Protein 6g

# Rosemary Potatoes

**Preparation Time:** 5 Minutes | **Cooking Time:** 5 Minutes | **Serves:** 2

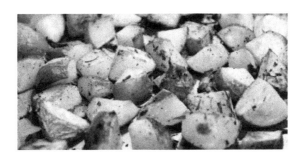

**Ingredients:**
- Three Large Red Potatoes, Cubed & Not Peeled
- 1 Tablespoon of Olive Oil
- Pinch Sea Salt
- ½ Teaspoon Rosemary, Dried

**Directions:**
1. Start by preheating your fryer to 390.
2. Combine your potatoes with olive oil, salt and rosemary. Make sure your potatoes are coated properly.
3. Cook for 5 minutes, and then check them. If you'd like them to be crispier than you can cook them for another two to three minutes.
4. You can serve them on their own or with sour cream.

Cal 150 | Fat 5g | Carb 9g| Protein 9g

# Olives, Green beans and Bacon

**Preparation Time:** 5 minutes | **Cooking Time:** 5 minutes | **Serves:** 4

**Ingredients:**
- ½ pound green beans, trimmed and halved
- 1 cup black olives, pitted and halved
- ¼ cup bacon, cooked and crumbled
- 1 tablespoon olive oil
- ¼ cup tomato sauce

**Directions:**
1. In a pan that fits the air fryer, combine all the ingredients, toss, put the pan in the air fryer and cook at 380°F for 5 minutes.

2. Divide between plates and serve.

Cal 160 | Fat 4g | Fiber 3g | Carb 5g | Protein 4g

## English Muffin Tuna Sandwiches

**Preparation Time**: 8 minutes | **Cooking Time**: 5 minutes | **Serves**: 4

**Ingredients**:
- 1 (6-ounce) can chunk light tuna, drained
- ¼ cup mayonnaise
- tablespoons mustard
- 1 tablespoon lemon juice
- green onions, minced
- English muffins, split with a fork
- tablespoons softened butter
- thin slices provolone or Muenster cheese

**Directions**:
1. In a small bowl, combine the tuna, mayonnaise, mustard, lemon juice, and green onions.
2. Butter the cut side of the English muffins. Grill butter-side up in the air fryer for 2 to 3 minutes or until light golden brown. Remove the muffins from the air fryer basket.
3. Top each muffin with one slice of cheese and return to your Kalorik Maxx Air Fryer. Grill for 2 to 3 minutes or until the cheese melts and starts to brown.
4. Remove the muffins from the air fryer, top with the tuna mixture, and serve.

Cal 389 | Fat 23g | Carb 25g | Fiber 3g | Protein 21g

## Cajun Shrimp

**Preparation Time**: 5 minutes | **Cooking Time**: 5 minutes | **Serves**: 6

**Ingredients**:
- Tiger shrimp (16-20/1.25 lb.)
- Olive oil (1 tbsp.)
- Old Bay seasoning (.5 tsp.)
- Smoked paprika (.25 tsp.)
- Cayenne pepper (.25 tsp.)

**Directions**:
1. Set the Air Fryer at 390º F.
2. Cover the shrimp using the oil and spices.

3. Toss them into your Kalorik Maxx Air Fryer basket and set the timer for 5 minutes.
4. Serve.

Cal 356 | Fat 18g | Carb 5g | Protein 34g

## Shrimp and Grilled Cheese Sandwiches

**Preparation Time**: 5 minutes | **Cooking Time**: 5 minutes | **Serves**: 4

**Ingredients**:

- 1¼ cups shredded Colby, Cheddar, or Havarti cheese
- 1 (6-ounce) can tiny shrimp, drained
- tablespoons mayonnaise
- tablespoons minced green onion
- slices whole grain or whole-wheat bread

tablespoons softened butt**Directions**:

1. In a medium bowl, combine the cheese, shrimp, mayonnaise, and green onion, and mix well.
2. Spread this mixture on two of the slices of bread. Top with the other slices of bread to make two sandwiches. Spread the sandwiches lightly with butter.
3. Grill in the air fryer for 5 to 7 minutes or until the bread is browned and crisp and the cheese is melted. Cut in half and serve warm.

Cal 276 | Fat 14g | Carb 16g | Fiber 2g | Protein 22g

## Simple Garlic Potatoes

**Preparation Time**: 5Minutes | **Cooking Time**: 5 Minutes | **Serves**: 2

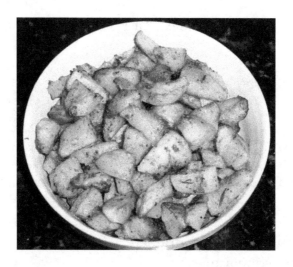

**Ingredients:**
- 3 Baking Potatoes, Large
- 2 Tablespoons Olive Oil
- 2 Tablespoons Garlic, Minced
- 1 Tablespoon Salt
- ½ Tablespoon Onion Powder

**Directions:**
1. Turn on your air fryer to 390.
2. Create holes in your potato, and then sprinkle it with oil and salt.
3. Mix your garlic and onion powder together, and then rub it on the potatoes evenly.
4. Put it into your air fryer basket, and then bake for 5 minutes.

Cal 160 | Fat 6g | Carb 9g | Protein 9g

## Flatbread

**Preparation Time:** 5 minutes | **Cooking Time:** 5 minutes | **Serves:** 2

**Ingredients:**
- 1 cup shredded mozzarella cheese
- ¼ cup almond flour
- 1-ounce full-fat cream cheese softened

**Directions:**
1. Melt mozzarella in the microwave for 30 seconds. Stir in almond flour until smooth.
2. Add cream cheese. Continue mixing until dough forms. Knead with wet hands if necessary.

3. Divide the dough into two pieces and roll out to ¼-inch thickness between two pieces of parchment.
4. Cover the air fryer basket with parchment and place the flatbreads into your Kalorik Maxx Air Fryer basket. Work in batches if necessary.
5. Cook at 320°F for 5 minutes. Flip once at the halfway mark.
6. Serve.

Cal 296 | Fat 22.6g | Carb 3.3g | Protein 16.3g

## Vegetable Egg Rolls

**Preparation Time:** 5 minutes | **Cooking Time**: 5 minutes | **Serves:** 8

**Ingredients:**
- ½ cup chopped mushrooms
- ½ cup grated carrots
- ½ cup chopped zucchini
- green onions, chopped
- tablespoons low-sodium soy sauce
- egg roll wrappers
- 1 tablespoon cornstarch
- 1 egg, beaten

**Directions:**
1 In a medium bowl, combine the mushrooms, carrots, zucchini, green onions, and soy sauce, and stir together.
2 Place the egg roll wrappers on a work surface. Top each with about 3 tablespoons of the vegetable mixture.
3 In a small bowl, combine the cornstarch and egg and mix well. Brush some of this mixture on the edges of the egg roll wrappers. Roll up the wrappers, enclosing the vegetable filling. Brush some of the egg mixture on the outside of the egg rolls to seal.
4 Air-fry for 5 minutes or until the egg rolls are brown and crunchy.

Cal 112| Fat 1g | Carb 21g| Fiber 1g | Protein 4g

## Hash Brown Burchett

**Preparation Time:** 5 minutes | **Cooking Time:** 5 minutes | **Serves:** 4

**Ingredients:**
- 4 frozen hash brown patties
- 1 tablespoon olive oil
- ⅓ cup chopped cherry tomatoes
- 3 tablespoons diced fresh mozzarella

- 2 tablespoons grated Parmesan cheese
- 1 tablespoon balsamic vinegar
- 1 tablespoon minced fresh basil

**Directions:**
1. Place the hash brown patties in the air fryer in a single layer. Air-fry for 5 minutes or until the potatoes are crisp, hot, and golden brown.
2. Meanwhile, combine the olive oil, tomatoes, mozzarella, Parmesan, vinegar, and basil in a small bowl. When the potatoes are done, carefully remove from the basket and arrange on a serving plate. Top with the tomato mixture and serve.

Cal 123 | Fat 6g | Carb 14g | Protein 5g

---

# Broccoli with Parmesan Cheese

**Preparation Time:** 5 minutes | **Cooking Time:** 4 minutes | **Serves:** 4

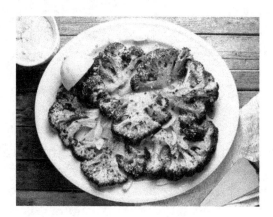

**Ingredients:**
- 1 pound broccoli florets
- 2 teaspoons minced garlic
- 2 tablespoons olive oil
- ¼ cup grated or shaved Parmesan cheese

**Directions**
1. Preparing the Ingredients. Preheat the air fryer to 360°F. In a bowl, mix together the broccoli florets, garlic, olive oil, and Parmesan cheese.
2. *Place the broccoli in the air fryer basket in a single layer and set the timer and steam for 4 minutes.*

Cal 130 | Fat 3g | Carb 5g | Protein 4g

# Cinnamon Pear Jam

**Preparation Time:** 5 minutes | **Cooking Time:** 4 minutes | **Serves:** 12

**Ingredients:**
- 8 pears, cored and cut into quarters
- 1 tsp cinnamon
- 1/4 cup apple juice
- 2 apples, peeled, cored and diced

**Directions:**
1. Put all of the ingredients in the air fryer and stir well.
2. Seal pot and cook on high for 4 minutes.
3. As soon as the cooking is done, let it release pressure naturally. Remove lid.
4. Blend pear apple mixture using an immersion blender until smooth.
5. Serve and enjoy.

Cal 103 | Protein 0.6g | Fat 0.3g | Carb 27.1g

# Yellow Squash Fritters

**Preparation Time:** 5 minutes | **Cooking Time:** 5 minutes | **Serves:** 4

**Ingredients:**
- 1 (3-ounce) package cream cheese, softened
- 1 egg, beaten
- ½ teaspoon dried oregano
- Pinch salt
- Freshly ground black pepper
- 1 medium yellow summer squash, grated
- ⅓ cup grated carrot
- ⅔ cup bread crumbs
- tablespoons olive oil

**Directions:**
1 In a medium bowl, combine the cream cheese, egg, oregano, and salt and pepper. Add the squash and carrot, and mix well. Stir in the breadcrumbs.
2 Form about 2 tablespoons of this mixture into a patty about ½ inch thick. Repeat with remaining mixture. Brush the fritters with olive oil.
3 Air-fry until crisp and golden, about 5 minutes.

Cal 234| Fat 17g | Carb 16g | Fiber 2g | Protein 6g

# Roasted Almonds

**Preparation Time: 5 minutes | Cooking Time:5 minutes | Serves: 8**

**Ingredients:**
- cups almonds
- 1/4 tsp pepper
- 1 tsp paprika
- 1 tbsp garlic powder
- 1 tbsp soy sauce

**Directions:**
1 Add pepper, paprika, garlic powder, and soy sauce in a bowl and stir well.
2 Add almonds and stir to coat.
3 Spray air fryer oven basket with cooking spray.
4 Add almonds in air fryer oven basket and cook for 5 minutes at 320°F..
5 Serve and enjoy.
Cal 143 | Fat 11.9g | Carb 6.2g | Sugar 1.3g | Protein 5.4 g

# Warm Peach Compote

**Preparation Time:** 5 minutes | **Cooking Time:** 1 minute/ **Serves:** 4

**Ingredients:**
- 4 peaches, peeled and chopped
- 1 tbsp water
- 1/2 tbsp cornstarch
- 1 tsp vanilla

**Directions:**
1. Add water, vanilla, and peaches into your Kalorik Maxx Air Fryer basket.
2. Seal pot and cook on high for 1 minute.
3. Once done, allow to release pressure naturally. Remove lid.
4. In a small bowl, whisk together 1 tablespoon of water and cornstarch and pour into the pot and stir well.
5. Serve and enjoy.
Cal 66 | Protein 1.4g | Fat 0.4g | Carb 15g

# Mushroom Pita Pizzas

**Preparation Time:5 minutes | Cooking Time: 5 minutes | Serves: 4**

**Ingredients:**
- (3-inch) pitas

- 1 tablespoon olive oil
- ¾ cup pizza sauce
- 1 (4-ounce) jar sliced mushrooms, drained
- ½ teaspoon dried basil
- green onions, minced
- 1 cup grated mozzarella or provolone cheese
- 1 cup sliced grape tomatoes

**Directions:**

1 Brush each piece of pita with oil and top with the pizza sauce.

2 Add the mushrooms and sprinkle with basil and green onions. Top with the grated cheese.

3 Bake for 5 minutes or until the cheese is melted and starts to brown. Top with the grape tomatoes and serve immediately.

Cal 231| Fat 9g | Carb 25g| Fiber 2g | Protein 13g

## Perfect Crab Dip

**Preparation Time:** 5 minutes | **Cooking Time**: 5 minutes | **Serves:** 4

**Ingredients:**

- 1 cup crabmeat
- 1 tbsp parsley, chopped
- 1 tbsp fresh lemon juice
- 1 tbsp hot sauce
- 1/2 cup green onion, sliced
- cups cheese, grated
- 1/4 cup mayonnaise
- 1/4 tsp pepper
- 1/2 tsp salt

**Directions:**

1 In a 6-inch dish, mix together crabmeat, hot sauce, cheese, mayo, pepper, and salt.

2 Place dish in air fryer oven basket and cook dip at 400°F for 5 minutes.

3 Remove dish from air fryer oven.

4 Drizzle dip with lemon juice and garnish with parsley.

5 Serve and enjoy.

Cal 313 | Fat 23.9g | Carb 8.8g | Sugar 3.1g | Protein 16.2g

## Honey Fruit Compote

**Preparation Time:**5 minutes | **Cooking Time:** 3 minutes | **Serves**: 4

**Ingredients:**

- 1/3 cup honey
- 1 1/2 cups blueberries
- 1 1/2 cups raspberries

**Directions:**
1 Put all of the ingredients in the air fryer basket and stir well.
2 Seal pot with lid and cook on high for 3 minutes.
3 Once done, allow to release pressure naturally. Remove lid.
4 Serve and enjoy.
Cal 141 | Protein 1g | Fat 0.5g | Carb 36.7g

# Air fried Bacon

**Preparation Time:** 1 minute | **Cooking Time**: 5 minutes | **Serves:** 6

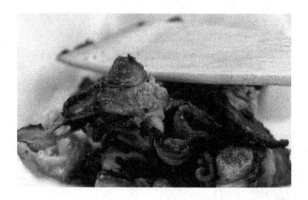

**Ingredients:**
- 6 bacon slices

**Directions:**
1. Place the bacon slices in air fryer oven basket.
2. Cook at 400°F for 5 minutes.
3. Serve and enjoy.

Cal 103 | Fat 7.9g | Carb 0.3g | Protein 7g

# Roasted Bananas

**Preparation Time:** 5 minutes | **Cooking Time:** 5 minutes | **Serves:** 2
**Ingredients:**

- 2 cups bananas, cubed
- 1 teaspoon avocado oil
- 1 tablespoon maple syrup
- 1 teaspoon brown sugar
- 1 cup almond milk

**Directions:**

1. Coat the banana cubes with oil and maple syrup.
2. Sprinkle with brown sugar.
3. Cook at 375 °F in the air fryer for 5 minutes.
4. Drizzle milk on top of the bananas before serving.

Cal 107 | Protein 1.3g | Fat 0.7g | Carb 27g

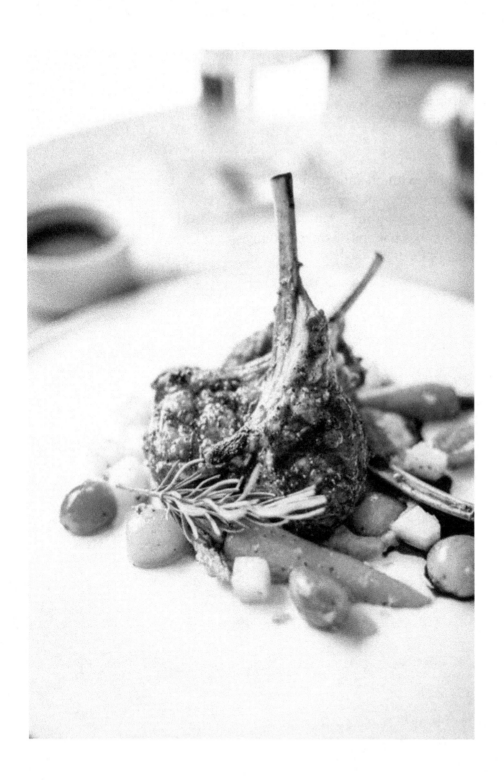

# Conclusion

The technology of the Kalorik Maxx Air Fryer Oven is exceptionally straightforward. Fried foods get their crunchy feel because warm oil heats meals quickly and evenly onto their face. Oil is a superb heat conductor that aids with simultaneous and fast cooking across each ingredient. For decades' cooks have employed convection ovens to attempt and mimic the effects of cooking or frying the entire surface of the food.

However, the atmosphere never circulates quickly enough to precisely attain that yummy surface most of us enjoy in fried foods. With this mechanism, the atmosphere is spread high levels up to 400°F, into "air fry" any foods like poultry, fish or processors, etc. This technology has altered the entire cooking notion by decreasing the fat by around 80 percent compared to traditional fat skillet. There is also an exhaust fan directly over the cooking room, which offers the meals necessary airflow.

This also contributes to precisely the identical heating reaching every region of the food that's being cooked. This is the only grill and exhaust fan that helps the Smart Oven improve the air continuously to cook wholesome meals without fat. The inner pressure strengthens the temperature, which will be controlled by the exhaust system. Exhaust enthusiast releases filtered additional air to cook the meals in a far healthier way. Smart Oven doesn't have any odor whatsoever, and It's benign, making it easy and environment-friendly.

Hopefully, after going through this cookbook and trying out a couple of recipes, you will get to understand the flexibility and utility of the air fryers. The use of this kitchen appliance ensures that the making of some of your favorite snacks and meals will be carried out in a stress-free manner without hassling around, which invariably legitimizes its worth and gives you value for your money.

We are so glad you leaped this healthier cooking format with us!

The air fryer truly is not a gadget that should stay on the shelf. Instead, take it out and give it a whirl when you are whipping up one of your tried-and-true recipes or if you are starting to get your feet wet with the air frying method.

Regardless of appliances, recipes, or dietary concerns, we hope you have fun in your kitchen. Between food preparation, cooking time, and then the cleanup, a lot of time is spent in this one room, so it should be as fun as possible.

This is just the start. There are no limits to working with the air fryer, and we will explore some more recipes as well. In addition to all the great options that we talked about before, you will find that there are tasty desserts that can make those sweet teeth in no time, and some great sauces and dressing to always be in control over the foods you eat. There are just so many options to choose from that it won't take long before you find a whole bunch of recipes to use, and before you start to wonder why you didn't get the air fryer so much sooner. There are so numerous things to admire about the air fryer, and it becomes an even better tool to use when you have the right recipes in place and can use them. And there are so many fantastic recipes that work well in the air fryer and can get dinner on the table in no time.

We are pleased that you pursue this Kalorik Maxx Air Fryer cookbook.